HOPE IN THE HARD PLACES

Journey Toward Healing Through Invisible Illness

Lynnette M. Wheeler

ISBN: 979-8-9949989-0-8

Cover design: Fairview Press Media Mgt.

Interior design: Lynnette M. Wheeler

Publisher: Guiding Lantern Press

Printed in the United States of America

For my husband, whose steady work, grounded strength, and tireless research made this possible.

For Greg, thank you for letting us be part of your journey.

And for Greg's family, who have carried more than anyone should have to. Your strength has not gone unnoticed.

TABLE OF CONTENTS

Preface

Every story begins somewhere, but Greg's began long before we understood it.

When I first sat down to write this book, my heart was full of emotions—hope, sadness, frustration, but above all, love. As Greg's mother, I have witnessed the impact of chronic illness and the confusion and pain that a misdiagnosis can bring. My motivation for sharing his story is to shine a light on the hidden struggles he endured and the strength that emerged when he refused to give up. This preface is both my tribute to Greg's resilience and a message of solidarity for others walking similar paths.

Covid-19 brought fear and uncertainty to families everywhere, but for Greg, the pandemic did more than disrupt routine; it triggered something deeper. The virus seemed to awaken underlying pathogens, making his symptoms more severe and unpredictable. What began as a global crisis soon became a personal one, forcing Greg to confront the possibility that his illness was more complex than he ever imagined.

By 2022, he battled symptoms that no one could explain. Doctors offered answers that didn't fit and treatments that failed to help. The search for the source of his suffering became a daily ritual, and with each new appointment, his hope wavered. The misdiagnoses meant more than missed opportunities for healing—they meant years spent in the dark, wondering what mystery illness was commandeering Greg's life.

My role as Greg's mom vacillated between comforter and advocate. I scoured articles, dug into research, listened to podcasts, questioned doctors and encouraged him to keep seeking. Sometimes, his dad and I could only offer support when his frustration boiled over or pain became unbearable. Other times, it meant pushing for answers when the system seemed to close its doors. Given that his dad and I live 3000 miles away, the journey has not been easy. We made it our mission to help Greg get diagnosed and treated by a doctor who understood him and what he was going through.

There were dark days for Greg, filled with anger at the illness, at the uncertainty, and the helplessness he felt. We mourned for him, the lost moments, and the life he deserved. But through perseverance, compassion, and the right guidance, we saw glimmers of hope. Each minor victory—

finding a compassionate doctor, receiving an accurate diagnosis, and beginning a promising treatment—became a reason to believe in a better future. Greg's courage in the face of pain was inspiring, reminding me that hope is not a luxury but a necessity.

Today, Greg looks to the future with cautious optimism. He dreams of simple joys: returning to his hobbies, rebuilding relationships, living a life not defined by illness. His goals, once clouded by uncertainty, are now guiding stars. As his mom, I am proud of the progress he has made and the hope he carries. His journey is not over, but he now walks it with more confidence and purpose.

To those reading this book—whether you are a patient, a parent, or someone seeking understanding—know that you are not alone. The path through chronic illness is often long and winding, but with love, advocacy, and hope, healing is possible. Greg's story is one of struggle, but also of resilience and triumph. May it inspire you to seek answers, provide support, and never lose sight of the future you dream for yourself or your loved ones.

This is where Greg's journey truly begins.

CHAPTER ONE

The Kitten in the Culvert

"Go deeper, Mom."

"I can't. The culvert is filling fast. I don't want to get stuck."

"Mom, I can still hear them. Just try."

I dropped to my stomach, cold mud soaking through my shirt, and reached into the black throat of the culvert. Water rushed past, icy and rising.

"I got one."

I couldn't see what I'd grabbed—only felt the frantic tremble of something tiny and terrified. All day, Greg and I had listened to the cries echoing under the road and watched the stray momma cat ferry her kittens into the shadows. She'd crossed the busy street again and again, babies dangling from her mouth, while we raked leaves on that crisp Halloween afternoon.

But now the tunnel was flooding, choked with debris, and the momma was gone.

Dusk swallowed the last bit of light. I handed the soaked kitten to Greg and slid forward again, inch by inch, letting sound guide me. The cries ahead were faint—thin threads unraveling in the water's roar.

I pushed deeper.

The water climbed.

The cries weakened. Then… nothing.

A silence so sudden it felt like the world stopped breathing.

I froze, listening, willing some small sound to return. When it didn't, I backed out, scraping my elbows on the concrete until I could stand. Rain hammered down, blurring everything.

Good. At least the rain would hide my tears.

The chorus of tiny voices that had haunted me all day was gone, swallowed by storm and darkness. I scanned the roadside for the momma cat, hoping for even a flicker of movement. Nothing.

Back home, we worked fast. We dried the trembling kitten, warmed him under a lamp, and mixed the formula we'd rushed to buy. The clerk had handed it over with a look that said he wasn't sure the little one would make it.

"Get him to a vet as soon as you can."

We named him Smokey. After a full belly, he burrowed into the blanket in his cardboard box with a weary trust that broke my heart. Our chocolate labs, Sadie and Sammy, stationed beside him like assigned guards.

The vet confirmed he was three weeks old—tiny, fragile, but a fighter. We'd never owned a cat; our home had always been full of dogs. But Smokey was different. Unexpected. Ours. And the beginning of something we didn't yet understand.

Greg was sixteen then, old enough to bond with Smokey before leaving for college. By that time, our once-rural road had grown busy and dangerous, so I tried to make Smokey an indoor cat.

Smokey disagreed.

The arrangement was uncomplicated: venture out by day and return at nightfall. Most of the time he honored it, but there were always exceptions—little escapades that turned into big worries.

Vacations were the worst. Smokey took personal offense at being left behind, slipping into the woods like a phantom. Sometimes he stayed gone for days. I'd stand at the edge of the yard at night, scanning the tree line for the glint of his iridescent eyes. When they finally appeared, my heart thudded with relief. He'd trot inside and leap onto Al's chest as if he hadn't vanished at all.

At least he was home, and I could breathe again.

When Smokey was three, he didn't come home one night. Nothing had changed. My nerves lit up. He sauntered in the next morning, unfazed, but by evening something was wrong. He was listless, crying, not eating. A swollen lump bulged on his shoulder.

At the vet, we learned he'd likely tangled with a raccoon. A puncture wound on the back of his neck—one I'd missed—had turned into a deep infection.

That was the start of an ordeal I wouldn't wish on anyone. Multiple surgeries. Sutures that wouldn't hold. Fluids everywhere. Smokey didn't care that he was sick; he wanted out and made sure we knew it.

After months of IV treatments and wrestling enormous antibiotic pills down his throat, the vet sat us down. Smokey might recover… or he might not. There were no guarantees.

I was exhausted. Smokey had decided I was the villain—the one who trapped him, medicated him, ruined his freedom. Al, of course, remained his favorite.

"No, we have to keep trying," Al said.

"Please." Half to him, half to fate.

We kept going.

After ten long months, Smokey recovered, but by then he'd worn me down—and most of our furniture with him.

"Out you go, Smokey. You've caused me enough grief for a lifetime."

His lifetime… and mine. I didn't know then how those words would circle back nearly twenty-five years later.

When he was thirteen, a tumor appeared on his neck—right where that old puncture wound had been. The vet removed it, and we were hopeful.

Six months later, the cancer returned—larger, angrier. Smokey had spent half a year fighting and never regained his spark. He was a wonderful companion, but it was time to let him go.

We mourned him deeply. His wild, loving nature made him unforgettable—equal parts chaos and devotion.

Something in the way he fought, survived, and kept returning from things that should have broken him stayed with us—quiet, insistent.

CHAPTER TWO

Building a Life

To understand Greg's story, you have to look back at the boy he once was—a child bursting with curiosity and creativity, always searching for meaning in the world around him. Nothing about him was passive; even his gifts had intention behind them. He didn't just absorb information—he took it in, turned it over in his mind until it became part of him. From the beginning, he was building himself piece by piece, long before any of us realized how much that would matter later.

Even in grade school, he learned faster than the lessons could keep up. Music came to him as naturally as breathing; he could pick up almost any instrument and make it sing. Greg's learning style always fascinated me. He listened with a kind of quiet intensity, taking in information once and holding onto it as if it had always belonged to him. When his dad showed him how to play the trumpet—an old horn from his own high-school days—Greg watched closely, nodded once, and lifted it to his lips. The first notes came out clear and confident. I tried afterward, but I couldn't push a single breath through the mouthpiece. Greg laughed, and his dad did too, while I handed the trumpet back and admitted I didn't have a musical bone in my body. Those two were naturals; I was clearly not.

By high school, when the academic material felt too familiar and he'd already mastered it, teachers often sent him to the music room—his favorite place to lose himself for an hour. While we introduced him to piano and violin in middle school, he taught himself brass and string instruments on his own, slipping easily from one to the next as if each one had been waiting for him.

His days were filled with skateboarding and snowboarding, his agility and daring a joy to watch. If there was a new skate park within a hundred-mile radius, he wanted to find it, and if there wasn't, he'd build his own ramps and rails in the driveway. He didn't just skate—he studied. I'd find him in the living room replaying Tony Hawk videos frame by frame, leaning his body in sync with the screen as if he could feel the physics through the carpet. Then he'd head outside and practice the same move over and over, falling, brushing himself off, trying again. By the time the neighborhood kids wandered over, he made it look easy, but I knew how many quiet hours of grit lived underneath those smooth landings.

He expressed himself through colorful clothes and wild hats that framed his long hair, a style that matched the brightness of his spirit.

Because his dad worked away as a merchant marine for long stretches of time, Greg and I developed a unique closeness. We were a bit of a duo—co-conspirators in fun—his boldness nudging awake the parts of me I'd tucked away long ago. I was his confidante and cheerleader as he built intricate Lego creations, his gentle, thoughtful nature shining through everything he touched. And in the winters, I'd occasionally liberate him from school and whisk him up to the Mt. Baker Ski Area for what I insisted were "field trips." He'd spend the afternoon polishing his snowboarding skills while I waited inside the lodge, drinking coffee and reading a good book. People loved to scold me for those absences, but Greg never missed a beat. Those days on the mountain taught both of us something—him about freedom, and me about the bright, colorful child I'd once been before I learned to dim my own light.

He had a steadiness that caught me off guard sometimes. Once, when I was shaken by a flat tire on a busy road, eight-year-old Greg noticed my hands trembling on the steering wheel. I admitted I didn't know how to change a tire, and he nodded like he'd already figured that out. "Let's just get out and wait," he said, matter-of-fact. "Someone will stop and help." And of course, he was right. A good Samaritan pulled over within minutes. Even after he developed Type 1 diabetes at age ten—a challenge he faced with quiet resilience—Greg remained funny, happy, and determined.

When Greg left home at eighteen, he moved into an apartment in town with a roommate, ready to begin his college years. Western Washington University felt familiar to him; he'd spent afternoons on that campus as a child while I worked toward my master's degree in psychology and counseling. He began college with two years of coursework already finished, yet he still didn't know what direction to take.

Engineering never sparked anything in him. He knew it. He felt it in his bones. He was going through the motions, doing what seemed practical, but it didn't light him up.

During that time, he worked full time at a senior retirement community. The residents adored the small group of young employees— Greg among them—treating them like adopted grandchildren. It was a grounding place for him, a pocket of warmth and purpose amid the uncertainty of early adulthood.

Eventually, Greg made a decision that surprised me. He told me he was applying to the Cordon Bleu College of Culinary Arts in Portland, Oregon.

"You want to be a cook?" I asked, trying to understand.

He didn't hesitate. "No, Mom—a chef."

It wasn't a whim. It was the first time I saw him choose something that felt entirely his. He loved the creativity, the precision, the way cooking blended art and science. And once he got there, he thrived—graduating at the top of his class in just two years.

Greg had always loved the science behind cooking, but it wasn't until culinary school that he realized how deeply it fascinated him. The chemistry, the structure, the way ingredients behaved under heat or pressure—it lit up the analytical part of his mind. Food science wasn't a childhood dream; it was something that took shape while he was immersed in the craft of cooking, something he recognized in himself as he grew more confident.

He knew he was capable. He never questioned that. What he didn't know was how to get from a culinary program to a scientific one. He just needed a pathway.

When one of his instructors pulled him aside and said, "You know, you'd be perfect for food science," it didn't plant a new idea. It simply named something Greg had already begun to feel. It was a moment of recognition—someone else seeing the direction he was already leaning toward. And that was enough to push him to take the next step.

He applied to Washington State University with a sense of purpose, believing he'd finally found the field that blended all the parts of him: creativity, curiosity, precision, and heart.

But WSU rejected him because of the chemistry grades he'd earned years earlier at WWU, during a time when he'd been drifting without direction. The letter hit him hard. Food science wasn't just an idea anymore—it was something he wanted. He sat at his small kitchen table, the rejection spread open in front of him, reading it over and over as if the words might change.

"I can't believe this," he said. "I know I can do this."

I told him he could try writing to the head of the Chemistry Department, but the decision to fight for it was his. He didn't want to let the younger version of himself close a door the older version was ready to walk through.

So he wrote—honestly, directly, in his own voice—and mailed the letter the next morning.

A few days later, my phone rang while I was at work. Greg's voice was tight, breathless.

"Mom—he called me."

The department chair had read his letter. He saw potential in Greg and offered provisional admission for one semester.

Greg didn't hesitate. He was ready to prove himself.

Once at WSU, Greg flourished. He built a strong relationship with the Chemistry chair—the same professor who had taken a chance on him. Their bond deepened over time, strengthened by something neither of them had expected: they were both Type 1 diabetics. It was an unspoken understanding, a shared vigilance, a quiet acknowledgment of the invisible calculations that shaped their days.

Over time, their relationship grew beyond that first connection. Greg earned the professor's respect through his work ethic and the way he approached problems—steady, curious, methodical. The professor became one of the most influential mentors in Greg's life, someone who recognized not just his potential, but the discipline and heart behind it.

Greg worked grueling early morning shifts, driving milk trucks at 4 a.m. from local farms to the university's cheese-making facility at Ferdinand's Creamery. One morning, during a blinding snowstorm, his tanker slid into a ditch. He called me because he knew I'd be awake—and because in moments like that, he always reached out to me. Eventually, another tanker arrived, the milk was transferred, and Greg continued on to the creamery. "Just another day at work," he said. I asked him to let me know when he was back safely. He always did.

When he came home for the holidays that year, he'd suddenly developed an allergy to Smokey. At the time it seemed minor, but looking back, it was the first hint that something inside him was beginning to shift.

After graduating from WSU with his food science degree, Greg built a solid career in quality assurance at various food manufacturing plants. He earned certifications, expanded his expertise, and carved out a life he was proud of. In 2009, he married his middle school sweetheart, Meagan, and the following year they welcomed their son, Murdoch.

Over the next decade, Greg moved through the familiar rhythms of adulthood—work, family, responsibility—but he always made room for creativity and adventure. He commuted to his job at Nature's Path on his motorcycle, a machine he tinkered with endlessly. He fabricated parts, upgraded components, and spent weekends riding through mountain roads and forest trails.

His creativity didn't stop there. On his wooden lathe, he turned out bowls and vases— smooth, elegant pieces that revealed an artist's patience. Two of his most remarkable creations, a handcrafted rocking chair and a matching bench, still sit proudly in his home. There was always something in Greg's creativity that felt familiar to me, a spark I recognized from a part of myself I hadn't visited in years.

During that same period, he took on a project that would have intimidated most people: refurbishing an old 20-by-40-foot chicken coop. The structure was weathered and sagging, but Greg saw possibility. He talked through each phase—raising the drooping walls, laying a new foundation, installing a sturdy floor—with the same confidence he brought to everything he touched.

"Please be careful, Greg. That building looks dangerous for one person to take on."

"Don't worry, Mom. I've designed a pulley system and jacks to help me. And I have the tractors. It's all under control."

And at that time, there was no reason not to believe him.

Before anything changed, before illness began to shadow his days, Greg was still chasing experiences that made him feel alive. In the fall of 2019, he went skydiving during a visit to see us in Florida. Meagan and Murdoch were with him, and together we waited for his turn. When he finally landed, he was practically glowing—his whole face lit up in a way I'd never seen.

Usually quiet by nature, he could barely get the words out fast enough. Being strapped to a professional skydiver had felt strange at first, every ounce of control handed over to a stranger he had to trust completely. At the open door of the plane, his legs trembled so hard the instructor must have felt it through the harness. Wind roared against him, a force so loud it filled his chest and made it hard to think.

And then they stepped out.

The world dropped away in a blur—air tearing past, the ground rushing up faster than thought. The instructor's weight pressed steady against his back as they fell together, the speed so intense it stole his breath. And then, just as suddenly, the chute opened and everything went quiet. The wind softened to a whisper. The horizon steadied. They drifted toward the earth in a kind of impossible stillness.

Seeing him that day—so full of color and fearlessness—stirred something in me, a version of myself I'd tucked away long ago.

He planned to return in the spring so we could jump together. A second jump within six months was half price, and he teased me about it until I finally agreed. I told myself there was plenty of time to come up with a good excuse to back out.

Back then, it felt like we had all the time in the world. Greg was healthy, thriving, and building a life he loved. None of us could see what was coming, or how quickly everything would shift when Covid arrived and the ground beneath all of us began to move.

He had built his life the same way he'd built himself—piece by piece, with intention and heart. That's what made what came next so devastating. Illness didn't just take his health; it reached into every piece he had worked so hard to create.

CHAPTER THREE

Covid Strikes

Greg flew to Florida alone in February 2020. He tried to convince Murdoch to come, but the long flight was a dealbreaker, so he came by himself, still buzzing from the skydive he'd taken months earlier. We never did the second jump he'd hoped for. Maybe I chickened out. Maybe the schedule was full. Maybe the place was closed, a victim of the Covid shutdowns. Neither of us remembers now. What mattered was that he'd already had that mile-high moment—the cold air slapping his face as the door opened, the weightless drop that stole his breath. A memory bright enough to carry him for years.

Life still felt ordinary then. Slow afternoons by the pool. Simple dinners out. Evenings with our longtime friends Lary and Deena, who had followed us from Washington to Florida years earlier. Greg had known them since he was young; being with them felt familiar and comfortable, like slipping into a well-worn rhythm.

While he was with us, the first case of Covid-19 appeared in Seattle. A headline, nothing more. The world around us looked unchanged—blue skies, crowded restaurants, people laughing over cocktails—so the news felt like a curiosity, not a warning. Not yet.

Florida seemed insulated, protected by distance and sunshine. Surely it wouldn't reach us. Surely it would stay on the other side of the country.

But when Greg flew home to WA in mid-February, the world he returned to was already tilting. He described shuttered storefronts, schools closing without notice, and offices going dark. Masks appearing everywhere. Lines snaking around grocery stores. A kind of nervous choreography taking shape—people stepping back, stepping aside, stepping away.

None of that had touched Florida. Not yet. And I clung to the illusion that it wouldn't.

Then I started watching the evening news again. I'd sworn off television months earlier to quiet my anxiety, but isolation has a way of pulling you toward the very things you try to avoid. Charts climbed. Predictions multiplied. Entire families fell ill after a single gathering. Numbers rose faster than the anchors could speak them.

The statistics came from national and global leaders, so they had to be accurate… right? Yet each night, certainty slipped a little further from reach.

Florida stayed calm until March 11th, when the World Health Organization declared a pandemic. The word hit like a dropped stone. Suddenly, our small community felt the tremor. The spring dance disappeared from the calendar. Tuesday coffee hour—gone. Entertainment nights—gone. The Canadian snowbirds packed their cars and fled north before the border closed behind them.

On March 13th, unable to reach Meagan, I texted Greg.

"I hope you guys are managing things okay… It's hard to know what's real, but it sure feels surreal. Love you, Mom."

Their world was tightening. Ours was simply growing quieter. We couldn't gather indoors, but we could still shuffle, play pickleball, ride our bikes. Outside felt safe. The pool allowed six people at a time, though most days it sat empty, the water still and waiting. A low hum of unease threaded through everything.

Greg texted back: "They set up a tent outside work. Temperature checks for everyone. If it's high, they send you home."

A new ritual. A new rule. A new way of moving through the world.

"How are Meagan and Murdoch?" I asked.

"Meagan's doing her best. At the girls' home it's just her and the kids most days. Murdoch's fine—he's been spending his days in his room, happy to have the quiet."

Our conversations shifted too. Less about hobbies or plans. More about outbreaks, predictions, and closures. The distance between us hadn't changed, but something in the tone had—a thin layer of worry settling over every exchange.

For the moment, we were all still standing. But the world was shifting beneath us, quietly at first, and none of us understood how deeply those shifts would reach.

In the early weeks after the declaration, we wandered through public spaces with masks tucked in our pockets, waiting to see what "normal" would become. I had a doctor's appointment scheduled for March 18th, but when I arrived, a paper sign hung crookedly on the clinic door: **ALL APPOINTMENTS CANCELED**

UNTIL FURTHER NOTICE. We hadn't even gotten a phone call. The office was dark. Doctors were transitioning to Skype appointments, a concept that felt more like science fiction than medicine.

My first telemedicine visit was on March 27th, and the experience was surreal. The screen cast a faint blue glare across my face, and the doctor's voice crackled through my laptop speakers, thin and metallic. At one point I found myself holding a thermometer up to the camera, angling it so she could read the numbers. How was a doctor supposed to check your vitals through a screen? Were they simply afraid to see patients face-to-face, or did they know something the rest of us didn't?

Only a few days later, on April 1st, the governor of Florida issued a two-week stay-at-home order—something many other states had already implemented or were preparing to.

Everyone began learning new ways to live. Groceries arrived at our door, and we washed everything, including the bags they came in. We learned to make our own masks and hand sanitizer because stores and online retailers had sold out. I sent Greg a picture of myself wearing the mask I'd sewn from one of his dad's red handkerchiefs.

"Remember when you couldn't wear a mask in a bank?" I asked.

"Yeah, insane, Mom. They would think you were going to rob the place."

A week later, I told Greg about the ambulance that came into the park to pick someone up. It was around 4 a.m. during my morning walk. At that hour, they didn't use sirens—they didn't want curious neighbors spilling out of their homes. I stood behind a palm tree in a neighbor's yard, watching the scene unfold. My heart was thumping wildly. It wasn't curiosity; it was terrifying.

"It was freaky, Greg. They looked like a SWAT team entering a meth lab—helmets, full-face breathing apparatuses, gloves, white hazmat suits."

I never found out what happened to Mary Sue. They whisked her away, and she never returned. I don't know whether she passed from the cancer she'd been battling or from Covid. She was simply gone, and the world was changing faster than any of us could make sense of.

Greg told me that in the food manufacturing industry, hand sanitizer had always been everywhere, even before Covid. But now the protocol was relentless. His dry, peeling hands were becoming painfully raw from the constant application of alcohol sanitizers.

"My hands are a mess, Mom. If I ever needed to be fingerprinted, they wouldn't be able to identify me. There're no grooves left. My hands feel like sandpaper."

"Wow, that's awful. Can't you use anything a little less harsh? Or just gloves?"

"Oh, we have to use gloves too. And the sanitizer is food regulation."

By then, most of the Canadians in our community had already headed home. Their government urged all citizens to return and quarantine, and many of our other snowbird neighbors left early as well.

We waited until May 8th, our usual migration date. We didn't know what to expect. The news was full of conflicting opinions about travel, shortages, and safety. Greg texted to check on our progress.

"What's it like out there, Mom?"

"Well, so far everything is great. We wear gloves everywhere, and I made a cleaning kit for the hotels—paper towels, alcohol wipes, antibacterial cleansers."

"How about gas?"

"We stop every chance we get, but the shortages we expected haven't happened. And there are hardly any commuters on the highway. Easy ride so far. It's just eerie."

"What about food?"

"I made sandwiches. Some stores are open, but I don't want to take any chances. And I wiped down everything in the hotel room—from the doorknob to the shower and sink fixtures. I even stripped the beds down to the clean sheets and used our own blankets and pillows."

We reached Maine in our usual three days and settled into our remote cabin on the lake. The ice had only just gone out, leaving the water dark and shockingly cold, a stillness that felt almost protective after the chaos we'd driven away from.

At night, the loons called across the cove, their long, wavering cries echoing through the pines and reminding us how far we were from anyone at all. The air smelled of wet earth and spruce, sharp and clean, and the isolation wrapped around us like a blanket—strange but comforting in a world suddenly full of danger.

Grocery deliveries weren't available, and stores were few and far between, so I had to figure out a new routine.

We adapted to the mask requirements and the limited capacity in larger stores. Walmart only allowed fifteen shoppers at a time, so the line stretched up and down the parking lot as everyone waited for their turn to enter. There wasn't much to choose from in rural Maine and the drive from the cabin to Walmart was 35 minutes, so if there was anything you wanted, you waited your turn. Social distancing markers appeared everywhere— six feet between shoppers, arrows on the floor dictating the direction of traffic. One afternoon, I told Greg about a fight that broke out in the grocery store.

"They have arrows on the floor showing which way to go, and someone was backing her cart up instead of moving forward. The woman behind her got irritated, and they had quite the exchange."

"You're gonna f'ing kill someone!" she yelled.

"Back off, b-tch!" the backward cart driver screamed.

"I was ahead of them at the end cap where Pepsi was on sale for $1.88 for a two-liter bottle. I remember it because I was pretending to study the price while watching them over my shoulder."

"Yes, it's happening here too, Mom," Greg said. "People feel frustrated and scared."

We had only a handful of neighbors scattered through the woods, but even among them, something subtle had shifted. People no longer stepped inside when they stopped by; they lingered on the porch steps or halfway down the drive, arms folded, bodies angled as if proximity itself carried risk.

One afternoon, a neighbor walked over to return a rake he'd borrowed. Before the pandemic, he would have come right up onto the porch, settled into one of the rocking chairs beside us, and we'd sit watching the loons or the boats on the lake, catching up on how everyone had fared through the winter months. This time was different.

He stopped several yards back, the rake held awkwardly in both hands, its long wooden handle wobbling as he tried to steady it. When he shifted his grip, the metal tines scraped against a rock, the sound sharp in the quiet afternoon. He gave a quick, nervous laugh and lifted the rake toward me like a fragile offering.

"Thought I'd bring this back," he said, his voice muffled behind the mask.

I stepped forward without thinking, the old instinct to greet and welcome rising before caution. The moment my foot touched the first porch step, he flinched—just a small recoil, barely a shuffle, but unmistakable. His shoulders tightened. His eyes flicked to the space between us as if measuring it.

"Oh—sorry," I said, stopping short.

"No, no, you're fine," he replied, though he took another half-step back, the rake still suspended between us like something dangerous or delicate.

We stood there for a beat, both of us pretending the distance wasn't loaded with fear. Eventually, I reached out and took the rake by the very end of the handle, careful not to brush his fingers. He nodded, already retreating down the drive, his wave stiff and apologetic.

It was such a small moment, but it told the truth none of us wanted to say out loud: something in the world had shifted, and even the simplest neighborly exchange now carried a tremor of unease.

Differing perspectives on safety measures, vaccinations, and crisis management had begun to reshape how people related to one another. Trust thinned. Some relationships fractured entirely. Fear simmered beneath the surface, and people displaced their anxiety onto anyone within reach.

"I figured something out about your dad," I told Greg one day.

"What's that, Mom?"

"We didn't realize how dependent he is on lip-reading. He's so deaf that even with his hearing aids, he doesn't notice when people are talking to him behind their masks."

"Well, apparently some states are allowing hearing-impaired people to go without masks because it's considered a disability."

"I didn't know that, Greg. But I don't think he wants to take that risk yet. Besides, someone would make a point of reminding you if you didn't have a mask on—or even if it wasn't fully covering your nose."

"Yes, there are plenty of people who feel it's their right or responsibility to tell you what the rules are. Or they make their own up."

We were back in our Florida home by October 2020, after another uneventful three-day drive along the coast. Soon after we settled in, Lary and Deena asked if I wanted to go to Washington with them in December. Just five days, they said, and we'd be home before Christmas.

"Really? Get on a plane? How would that even work?

Deena shifted in her seat, not quite meeting my eyes. She wasn't terrified, just… hesitant. Ever since the pandemic began, she'd been careful about everything—more sensitive to risk than most, thoughtful about every decision. The idea of flying made her uneasy, though she tried not to show it.

Lary, meanwhile, was the opposite. He waved a hand as if Covid were more of a nuisance than a threat.

"They've got all their safety protocols in place—limited passengers, lots of empty seats, masks," he said, full of his usual confidence. But there was a softness under it, a kind of practiced steadiness. He wasn't shrugging off the risks so much as trying to shoulder the worry for the rest of us, especially Deena. His confidence was less bravado than reassurance, a way of saying *we'll get through this together*. "We'll be fine."

"Well, let me check with Greg and see if he thinks it's a good idea."

Greg talked it over with Meagan, and they thought it would be okay, so I bought the ticket. Deena still looked a little unsure, but she trusted Lary's optimism. I just wanted to see Greg and his family for a couple of days. Something in me sensed life was about to get even stranger.

But in early December, Greg called.

"Mom, I think you should wait. Something about traveling right now just feels wrong."

The familiar tug pulled at me—wanting to see him, wanting him safe.

The airline refunded my ticket without a fuss.

"Okay," I said, trying to sound lighter than I felt. "Maybe things will calm down soon."

He exhaled, a sound more weary than worried. "I'm not sure they will, Mom. Not for a while."

His words stayed with me. Even as life in Florida carried on in its quiet, cautious way, a thin thread of unease wound itself through my days.

A few of my neighbors contracted Covid over the holidays, and their experiences were touch and go. Whether hospitalized or isolated at home, the loneliness of fighting it alone was traumatic.

Greg and I talked about it often. He knew many of our Florida friends, and he shared what was happening at his workplace—people getting sick, morale plummeting, employees quitting or simply not showing up. I told him about Bill and Dotty, the first Covid cases in our park.

"Bill's fighting this in the hospital, and he's in awful shape. Dotty's home alone, and none of us can visit. We leave food on her doorstep, ring the bell, and walk away."

What I didn't say was how strange and heartbreaking that ritual had become. You'd set the casserole or the bag of groceries down, step back to the end of the driveway, and wait—hoping she'd come to the door, hoping she felt well enough to take what you'd brought. Sometimes she'd appear in the doorway, small and tired, and give the faintest wave. That tiny gesture was the only proof she was still fighting.

"That's horrible," Greg said.

And then there was Bill. He survived his hospital ordeal, but when the ambulance brought him home, we stood outside and watched as they stopped at the end of his driveway. The paramedics were covered head to toe in protective gear. Bill had to walk the whole length of the driveway alone, unsteady but determined, while they tossed his clothes and belongings from the ambulance into his front yard as if they were still radioactive. It was surreal, almost cruel, but that was the world we were living in—everyone terrified of getting too close.

They both survived, but not without consequences. Bill lost thirty-five pounds and battled long Covid for over a year. He was afraid to tell anyone—he kept testing positive for months, even though he felt fine, and no one really knew what to make of that yet. Dotty faced ongoing heart issues and a weakened immune system.

Thankfully, Lary and Deena made it back to Florida safely. None of us went out much anymore. We relied on the safety of outdoor visits under our covered patio, spaced chairs and soft evening breezes replacing the closeness we once took for granted. We even had a few birthday celebrations—minus the candles, because blowing them out suddenly felt dangerous.

One afternoon, we had Greg on speakerphone.

"You've got to be careful, Greg. With your diabetes, you're at high risk."

"I know, Mom. But there's not much I can do except be safety smart."

"Just live a little, Greg," Lary chimed in. His voice had that familiar lift to it, the kind he used whenever the rest of us were teetering on the edge of worry. "When are you coming back to Florida?"

"Not sure. Maybe if they get that vaccine finished."

His voice carried a mix of hope and hesitation—an uncertainty we all felt but rarely admitted. For a moment, Lary went quiet, the kind of pause that didn't happen often with him. When he spoke again, the bravado softened, replaced by something steadier, almost gentle.

"Your mom misses you."

It wasn't loud or showy, just a small truth offered into the space between us. His confidence wasn't about pretending everything was fine; it was his way of holding the rest of us up, giving us something solid to lean on when the world felt anything but.

CHAPTER FOUR

The Year the Ground Shifted—2021

When the vaccine became available, essential professions were first in line—medical personnel and first responders. Those working in the food manufacturing industry became eligible on March 17, 2021, and Greg scheduled his first appointment three days later.

His father and I, labeled "elderly" and therefore high-risk, had already made it through the system. Greg received his second shot on April 17th and woke the next day with severe side effects—head and neck pain, along with deep, aching fatigue. Many of us had complained of headaches and malaise after our shots, so we assumed his reaction was part of the process.

A few days later, Greg boarded a plane to Florida to spend a couple of weeks with us. He hadn't visited in a year, and for Murdoch it had been even longer—over eighteen months. There were still restrictions in place, but Greg needed his bi-yearly dose of sunshine. Washington averages nearly 190 days of measurable rain each year, and the weight of the pandemic had worn all of us thin. He was willing to take his chances.

And besides, I still cut his hair—and he hadn't had a trim in over a year. It had grown down to his neck, thick and uneven, with new streaks of gray and silver that hadn't been there the last time I saw him. I didn't know if it was stress, illness, or just the year we'd all lived through, but it startled me a little. He kept most of it tucked under a ballcap, pulled low the way he always wore it, but once he took it off, the overgrowth was impossible to miss.

We set up outside in the sunshine. Greg sat shirtless in a lawn chair, and as I worked, the clippings drifted down onto his hairy chest—short dark curls mixed with the new silver. I started with the trimmers, buzzing a clean line from the back of his neck forward, the vibration steady in my hand. I'd been cutting his hair since he was a kid, but after a year apart, I felt strangely nervous, wanting to get it just right.

He kept laughing, telling me to relax, telling me he trusted me, which only made me more determined not to mess it up. Once the bulk was off, I switched to scissors, shaping and smoothing until the familiar version of him emerged again. And then, right on cue, the little cowlick at the crown of his head popped back up—something I hadn't seen in so long it made me smile, a tiny reminder of the boy he used to be.

When I finally stepped back, he ran a hand through the shorter layers and grinned.

He looked great. And for a moment, standing there in the warm Florida sun with hair clippings scattered around us, life felt almost normal again.

Despite the lingering pandemic rules, we enjoyed ourselves. Masks were required everywhere, but that didn't stop us from eating out, shopping, or visiting our favorite theme parks. Murdoch lived in the pool that year. I took several videos of him racing the length of the water against Rico, a seventy-year-old man who was still impressively fit. Murdoch always won, though I suspect Rico may have given him a generous head start. Greg and I cheered from the sidelines, soaking in the simple joy of it.

After those intense pool marathons, Murdoch always wanted fruit.

"Grandma, can you take me to the fruit stand? I want to get some dragon fruit."

"Yeah, let's go," I said. "They have the best Amish cheese there too."

Seeing them again after such a long separation felt like a gift. We hoped the worst was behind us—that life might settle into something resembling normal again, and we could resume our twice-yearly visits. There was still uncertainty, but we promised ourselves we'd make it happen if the world would just steady itself a little longer.

At the end of May, on my way to Maine for the summer, Greg and I were texting. Out of nowhere, he asked, "Mom, have you ever heard of depersonalization or derealization?"

The words caught me off guard. I knew them vaguely from my years as a therapist, but it had been so long that I had to look them up again just to be sure I remembered correctly.

"What's going on?" I asked.

"I don't know," he wrote. "It's like… I feel outside myself sometimes. Like I'm watching my life instead of living it. Everything feels a little foggy, a little unreal."

He paused, then added, "There's something going on in my head. It's a weird sensation."

He said he wondered if he had a "mild case," though he wasn't sure what that meant. The conversation unsettled me. Greg had always been introspective, always researching things that caught his attention, but something about the way he described it felt different.

"I take a lot of risks in life and have thoughts of death and dying," he said next. "Is that normal, Mom?"

I slipped into therapist mode without meaning to. Even after eight years of retirement, the instinct was still there. To be honest, the therapist in me stepped forward because the mother in me was afraid. I listened carefully, asked questions, and tried to understand what he was really saying.

The more we talked, the more I felt he didn't meet the criteria for anything clinical. I reminded myself that high-risk activities can trigger endorphins, the brain's natural 'feel good' chemicals, and Greg had always chased that sense of aliveness. And with the news cycle predicting thousands of deaths each week, I knew it wasn't unusual for thoughts about mortality to surface.

He assured me he wasn't suicidal—just curious. Curious about dying, about what it meant, about why the idea kept floating through his mind.

I told him that skydiving and riding a motorcycle didn't mean he had a death wish. They were just things that made him feel awake in a world that had gone numb.

"Thanks for coming out of retirement and listening, Mom," he said. "I needed a therapy session this afternoon."

"Yeah, anytime, Greg. I'm glad you still feel comfortable talking to me about your feelings."

It made me smile that my middle-aged son still trusted me with his deepest thoughts. But after we hung up, the conversation lingered. Something about it felt different, and I couldn't quite name why.

It was only in retrospect that I wondered if he was experiencing the earliest shifts—subtle changes neither of us yet understood.

Murdoch and Meagan came to Maine for a summer vacation in August. They explored the state on their own, and we spent long, warm days boating, tubing, and paddleboarding on the lake. We all put puzzles together on the kitchen table late into the evenings. We took a trip to the coast to visit Al's sister, Sharon, and her husband, Arthur, where we played pool and putt-putt golf on Arthur's whimsical 18-hole course. It wound through trees and quirky obstacles—water holes, tunnels, ramps, even windmills. Murdoch took to it immediately, lining up each shot with a seriousness that made all of us laugh, and somehow sinking the impossible ones.

He tried his first Maine lobster and loved it. Arthur took him on a tour of Islesboro in his golf cart, and the two of them bonded in that easy way children and kindhearted adults sometimes do. Greg was missing out, but we talked to him every day.

Two months later, in October 2021, Greg and Murdoch traveled to Florida for two weeks. We had a wonderful time—exploring, eating out, cooking at home, swimming, and riding roller coasters. Well, they rode the roller coasters. I got dizzy just watching from the ground.

Greg mentioned he'd been having a lot of joint pain and muscle aches, but we brushed it off. We'd been doing more physical activity than he was used to. We also rented a beach house on Anna Maria Island for a few days. The weather was perfect; the sand velvety soft; the water cool and invigorating. It felt like a small return to normal.

When they flew home to Washington, I assumed life would settle back into its usual rhythm for all of us. I slipped easily into mine— pickleball in the afternoon, planning holiday events for our community, organizing the upcoming social season. Florida was easing into its best weather of the year, and my days felt light, predictable, almost carefree. If anything was wrong in Washington, I didn't know it. Greg didn't mention anything beyond the usual busyness of work and parenting, and I didn't press. Why would I? Everything seemed fine.

But while I was moving through my sunny routines, Murdoch wasn't feeling well. For weeks he'd been unusually tired, drinking water constantly, and losing weight—changes no one wants to see in an eleven-year-old. I didn't know any of this at the time. I was living my life in Florida; they were managing theirs in Washington.

At the beginning of December, Greg called.

"Mom, I have something to tell you."

"What's going on, Greg?"

"Murdoch's at Children's Hospital in Seattle. You know he hasn't been feeling well."

"Yes, you've told me. What's wrong?"

"He has Type 1 diabetes."

"No," I cried. "It was supposed to skip his generation. I'm so sorry."

My mind flashed back to Greg at age ten—exhausted and thirsty—the same symptoms now showing up in his son.

"Mom, he's fine and in good spirits. We're all doing the diabetes class together, but he won't have to stay long since I know what to do."

His diagnosis devastated me. Even with insulin and careful monitoring, the disease makes a child's life harder. We had tried to make Greg's life as normal as possible, yet he still faced challenges—not only from peers but from adults who didn't understand the condition.

Now Murdoch would have to navigate those same hardships, on top of the chaos and uncertainty his generation was already facing.

It was not a great way to end the year.

I didn't know it then, but 2021 was the year the ground quietly shifted beneath us. The years that followed would show us just how much.

CHAPTER FIVE

Medical Malaise 2022—2024

In early 2022, a small shift in Greg's voice told me something was wrong. He mentioned his eyes before anything else. "My vision's been giving me trouble," he said. "The ophthalmologist wants to start injections."

He tried to sound casual, but the strain in his voice was unmistakable. The words landed with a weight I couldn't ignore. Eye injections. Needles. No anesthesia. Even he couldn't hide how much it unnerved him.

Only a few weeks earlier, life had felt almost normal again. In March 2022, he and Murdoch had flown to Florida, and for the first time since the pandemic, travel felt easy. Murdoch had adapted to his diabetes with surprising grace—swimming, biking, challenging anyone who'd play 8-ball on our community pool table. For a moment, we'd all believed the worst was behind us.

But Greg's vision kept slipping. When his eyes began to hemorrhage, the mask he'd been wearing cracked. The diagnosis—diabetic retinopathy—shouldn't have surprised us. He'd lived with Type

1 diabetes since childhood. Yet the speed of the decline didn't sit right with him. Something felt off, as if this was only the beginning of a much larger unraveling.

Looking back, that was the moment the picture blurred, the way his vision had—clear one day, slipping the next.

As the autumn leaves began to change, a restlessness settled into Greg's voice.

"I just don't feel well," he said. "My whole body hurts. I've been reading about different things people experience after vaccines. Do you know anything about that, Mom?"

"No, Greg. I haven't read anything about it, but I'll look into it."

He hinted at things he wasn't telling us, offering only fragments—just enough to acknowledge something was wrong, never enough to reveal its weight.

A few weeks later, he and Murdoch flew to Florida in late October 2022. We all dressed up for the Halloween party at our community clubhouse—me in a pink wig and poodle skirt, Murdoch in his tie-dyed hippie outfit with a bandana and dark glasses. With his long, beautiful hair flowing down his back, he looked like he'd stepped straight out of the 60s.

I was having a wonderful time, but Greg seemed quieter than usual. So quiet that I don't remember what he wore for a costume. He was not obviously ill—just… muted. His laughter lagged behind the moment, like he had to reach for it. He drifted at the edges of conversations, watching more than participating. When I tried to pull him into a photo, he shook his head with a tired smile and slipped away. At the time, I told myself he was worn out from travel, but a small, persistent tug pulled at me, something I couldn't quite name.

When they returned in the spring of 2023, that tug had grown heavier. Greg moved through the days as if he were carrying a private burden he couldn't set down. His joint pain had worsened, and the fatigue settled over him the way morning mist drifts across the lake—thin at first glance, but impossible to ignore once you see it. There was a subtle cognitive fog too—tiny hesitations, misplaced words, moments when his eyes went distant before he snapped back with a joke. The humor was still there, but it felt like a thin layer stretched over something deeper.

One afternoon he sat down beside me, slower than usual. "My bones hurt, Mom," he said.

The quiet in his voice did more than the words themselves. It opened something raw inside me.

"Wow," I said softly. "That's not good."

He lifted his shirt almost casually, as if it were nothing, and showed us something he'd never mentioned before—thick, dark purple lesions running across his skin. Not stretch marks. Not really. These were deeper, angrier, the color of bruises that refused to fade.

"They showed up when I was a teenager," he said. "Sometimes they flare. Get darker. Itchy. Burning."

The words were light, almost tossed off, but his eyes didn't match his voice. He wouldn't look at me. That small avoidance said more than any confession could.

"So they change?" I asked.

"Yeah. Sometimes lighter. Sometimes like this."

He shrugged, but the shrug felt practiced, like something he'd rehearsed to make the truth seem smaller. And suddenly everything—his pain and fatigue, the vision problems, now this—stacked together in a way that made my chest tighten. Something was wrong. Not just diabetes-wrong. Deeper-wrong.

I thought of my own stretch marks from pregnancy, how they'd softened into pale threads over the years. Greg's had been there for more than two decades. They should have faded by now, but they hadn't. If anything, they were getting worse.

Why? Why are they still so dark?

He'd always been a slim teenager, steady, never the kind of kid whose body changed enough to leave marks like these. And sitting beside him now, watching him try to shrug off something that clearly frightened him, a quiet ache gathered in me, the kind that rises before the mind can explain it.

Greg traveled to Maine alone that September, saying he needed a break from everything. Struggle clung to him, even if he couldn't explain it. His movements had slowed; his speech came out in a pressured cadence. Something heavy sat on him, unnamed but unmistakable.

At the lakefront cabin, we tried to pretend life was simple again—boating, relaxing, lingering on the porch as if normalcy could be willed into existence.

Then Hurricane Lee swept through, dragging a tornado behind it that ripped out trees and shattered docks around the lake. The sky darkened with a kind of abruptness that matched the pressured cadence in Greg's voice these days, the wind rising with a restless, unpredictable energy that reminded me of him.

Our dock was barely holding on. Greg plunged into the torrential rain with his father, fighting the storm as if he could muscle the chaos back into place. Rain lashed sideways. The wind howled. Greg braced himself against it, gripping the boards, refusing to let the dock break loose. He lifted the sledgehammer over his head and slammed it down, trying to drive the posts deeper into the lake bottom as the dock rocked beneath him. Determination radiated off him—fierce, almost defiant—as though wrestling the storm might quiet whatever turmoil churned inside him.

Another one of those risk-taking moments that made him feel alive. Or maybe something else entirely—a need to push back against whatever was pulling at him.

When the storm finally passed, the waves calmed and sunlight returned, but Greg didn't. Having him with us was wonderful, yet his energy never lifted. He moved through the days with a deep introspection, a dimming I couldn't ignore. The light in him flickered like the power lines after the storm—present, but unsteady.

I tried to tease out the humor that always made me laugh, but it wouldn't come. My own laughter felt thin when he mentioned his aches and pains.

"Ah, you're just getting old, Greg," I joked.

Inside, the words scraped against something that refused to agree. That can't be. He's in the prime of his life. Later, I worried he might have heard it as me minimizing his pain. I only meant to keep things light, but something in me already knew this wasn't just "getting old."

Back home in Everson, Washington on Halloween night, Greg suffered a massive orbital hemorrhage and lost much of his vision. He didn't tell us for weeks. When he finally did, his voice sounded distant, almost hollow, as if he were describing someone else's crisis. The worst part was the doctors' confusion. No one could explain why it had happened.

Our last visit from Greg and our grandson came in February 2024. Only now do I see how close we were to the edge—how tightly he was holding himself together just long enough to make the trip. He kept brushing off his symptoms, offering reassurances that thinned each time he spoke them.

Seeing them that week thrilled me. I hoped the Florida sunshine might lift them both. We did our usual outings to Busch Gardens and SeaWorld. They rode roller coasters while I watched from below. Even from a distance, something in Greg's posture was off—the way he braced before each ride, the way he moved afterward as if every joint protested.

By evening, exhaustion clung to him. One night his headache was so severe he collapsed onto the bed fully clothed, shoes still on. The sight of him lying there like that sent a cold ripple through me.

"I've known people with Type 1 who developed rheumatoid arthritis," I said softly. "When you get home, have a rheumatologist take a look."

"Okay, Mom. I will."

The words came out thin, drained of conviction, as if even promising was too much.

I wasn't doing well myself that spring. A back injury from the fall before, then months of respiratory infections—sinusitis, bronchitis, pneumonia. After sinus surgery in April, I finally emerged from the fog I'd been living in. My illnesses had names. Greg's didn't. His health kept slipping, and he withdrew further, calling less often. Each silence felt heavier than the last.

I kept reaching out.

"What are you doing for the pain?"

Even before he answered, I sensed the shift. February had been the last time he could pretend things were manageable. Something had turned in him on that trip—subtle, irreversible—settling between us like a shadow neither of us could name.

He tried everything he could think of: a TENS unit, microdosing mushrooms, acupuncture.

"The TENS unit distracts me for a little while," he said.

"And the mushrooms?"

"Maybe a slight difference. Hard to tell. The dose is tiny. No negatives so far."

Acupuncture brought brief, inconsistent relief—like catching his breath for a moment before sinking back under.

By August, his symptoms were overwhelming. He asked his doctor for a specialist referral. In September, the rheumatologist ruled out rheumatoid arthritis but offered nothing else.

His eyes were worsening too. The injections weren't helping, so the ophthalmologist suggested stepping up treatment with retinal laser photocoagulation—tiny burns on the retina to seal leaking vessels.

By October 2024, Greg had undergone eight eye surgeries. His frustration was boiling over.

"I feel like my head is going to explode," he said. "It's like someone is poking hot daggers into my eyeballs."

Still, he drove himself to and from work because, as he put it, "I have to." Nature's Path was forty minutes away along rural roads. He refused to drive in the dark or toward Bellingham, the largest hub in the community.

"Too risky," he said. "Too much traffic. My eyes are getting worse."

His wife took time off work to drive him to appointments when he needed to go into town.

In December, he saw an Ear, Nose, and Throat specialist (ENT) for the crushing headache that had been building for weeks. The doctor prescribed a Z-pack and prednisone, admitting he didn't see an infection and didn't know what was wrong. He ordered a CT scan, but the earliest appointment was mid-January.

Looking back, it's hard to believe how many specialists he saw without anyone truly seeing him. Each appointment ended the same way—more waiting, more dismissal, more doors quietly closing.

A week passed. Greg couldn't wait. The pain was unbearable.

"I have so much pressure in my head," he said. "I can't take this."

On New Year's Eve, I was at a dance in our community clubhouse. A knot of anxiety sat in my chest, making it impossible to enjoy the night. Greg was in the Emergency Room (ER), where he'd spent most of the day waiting. My son was desperate for answers, and no one seemed able to help.

At 8:42 p.m., my phone buzzed.

"Two different CT scans show nothing. Sent me home with a Percocet. I'm very frustrated."

"Percocet isn't much of a solution," I wrote back. "Did they recommend a neurologist? And what about your vision?"

"I don't know, Mom. Even though I can hardly see, the eye doctor says I'm good. This was the least helpful experience I've ever had in my life."

"I'm so sorry, Greg. Let's talk tomorrow. Try to get some rest."

I left the dance early and cried the night into the next year. While everyone else celebrated the arrival of 2025, I prayed for something— anything—to change for Greg. For someone to listen. For someone to help.

He felt defeated, unheard, dismissed, angry. And all I could do was watch as my son slipped deeper into a world of pain no one could explain. As 2025 began, I had no idea how quickly everything was about to unravel.

CHAPTER SIX

The Unraveling—2025

The next day, Greg opened the ER notes from his visit the night before. It didn't take long for panic to set in. He called me almost immediately, and the moment I heard his voice, it was clear the night's reassurance hadn't lasted.

"How's your headache?" I asked. "You said the CT scan showed nothing."

"It's horrible. It doesn't quit. And one of the CT scans *did* show something—a four-millimeter hyperdense nodule. The radiologist thinks it might be a small meningioma. He wants an outpatient MRI with contrast. The ER doctor didn't care. He brushed it off. Said it was all in my head."

"It is in my head!" he yelled. "I have a brain tumor."

He was spiraling, and I could hear the fear in his voice, that sharp edge that told me he was slipping into a place where reason couldn't reach him.

"If you don't have active head trauma or a brain hemorrhage, they don't treat it as an emergency," he said, his tone hardening. "I figured that out by going through the test results myself. Nobody tells you anything."

We stayed on the phone, talking through his anger and frustration, trying to shift the conversation toward next steps. Eventually he settled enough to think more clearly. It was the weekend, and there wasn't much he could do except research and wait—two things that only fed his anxiety.

On Monday, he called his primary care doctor and asked for a referral. They scheduled the MRI for Friday. His pain was unbearable, so he took the week off work to decide what to do after the scan, giving himself space to breathe and gather whatever strength he had left. His anxiety was sky high, so he asked for something to help him get through the procedure. The doctor prescribed a single dose of lorazepam.

Convinced he had a brain tumor, Greg spent the week researching neurosurgeons, diving into medical websites and patient reviews as if the right specialist might hold the key to saving his life. On Wednesday, he texted me:

"There's a state-of-the-art gamma knife neurosurgery center in Orlando. Really highly rated."

"What about Seattle?" I asked.

Maybe he wanted to be closer to us. Maybe he was grasping for any sense of control. I wasn't sure.

"I'll look into it," I told him. "But first you'll need to see what the MRI shows and what the doctors recommend."

"Yes. I know, Mom."

Friday arrived, and Greg was waiting for the procedure. I asked if Meagan was with him, hoping he wasn't alone. She had gone to pick Murdoch up from school and would return later.

"I'm in the waiting room," he said. "They're doing an MRI with and without contrast."

His voice was steady, softened by the medication they'd given him, and for a moment I let myself believe he might finally be getting a small measure of relief.

After it was over, he texted me.

"All done, Mom. Now we wait. They were really thorough. The tech said they got great images—whatever that means."

"Okay, thank you, Greg. Get some rest, and I'll talk to you tomorrow."

The next morning, I heard from Meagan. She sounded exhausted and frustrated, the kind of worn-down fatigue that comes from carrying too much for too long without a break. Greg was having a meltdown—not because he had a tumor, but because he didn't. The absence of an answer felt like another blow.

I didn't see any of their day-to-day life during this time. What I knew came in fragments—a phone call here, a text there—pieces of a marriage under pressure that I could only glimpse from the outside. Meagan was carrying more than anyone should have to, and although she wasn't always physically present with Greg, I could hear in her voice how worn down she was.

"Greg needs his dad," she said.

"Should we come right now?" Meagan paused. "No. Not yet."

I could hear the strain in her voice, the weight she was carrying. I didn't push.

"Okay," I said. "I'll look for tickets, and we can talk about it later."

She opened up about how Greg's illness had affected her and Murdoch. His erratic emotions had created a chasm between them. She was juggling work, graduate school, parenting, and Greg's escalating needs—all without a roadmap, and certainly without the support anyone would need to navigate that kind of emotional terrain.

"Has he been abusive?" I asked quietly. She hesitated. "No… but he yells at the dogs."

"He's projecting his frustration," I said. "I'm sorry you're going through this. We'll try to help however we can."

"Thanks. I just… I can't do the medical stuff right now. I don't have it in me."

"We'll do what we can, Meagan. You focus on what you need to."

I called Greg and asked him to send me the MRI results, then talked him down again. Although he was convinced he had a tumor, the doctors had ruled that out. "There has to be a tumor," he said. "I can feel it." Still, other conditions—things like increased intracranial pressure—could cause symptoms like his.

I had already done my research because I could see where his mind was going. He was desperate for a resolution, and I wanted him to know we believed him. Something was happening. They just hadn't found it yet.

"I'm sorry you're going through this, Greg. We're here to support you while you work through it, and we'll stay with you step by step, no matter how long it takes. Keep searching for answers; you're making progress and have eliminated several possibilities. We love you."

I offered to get him a good HEPA filtration unit for his bedroom. He thought it might help him breathe more easily. It was midweek, and he still hadn't heard from his doctor, so he felt ignored—left to figure everything out on his own.

"I'm going to request a blood test for toxoplasmosis tomorrow," he said. "I was working with a lot of dirt and soil last spring."

"What's that?"

"Toxoplasmosis. It's a parasite—you can get it from cat feces or contaminated soil. Since I handled so much dirt last spring resurrecting the chicken coop, I want to rule it out."

"Okay, Greg. Is there anything else you can think of?"

"I'm going to ask for a second referral to see another ophthalmologist."

"Good idea."

"And I'm still waiting for an appointment with a neurologist." There was a pause—long enough for me to feel it.

"Also… I can't work, so I'm requesting time off under the Family and Medical Leave Act."

"I understand, Greg, and we support you. It's been a full-time job trying to figure out what's wrong."

There was a quiet tension beneath everything that winter, a financial undercurrent we rarely spoke aloud. When Greg decided to take family leave in January 2025, we all felt the weight of it. We wanted him to rest, to heal, but we also worried about how the sudden loss of income might affect them. They had always managed their mortgage responsibly—we had only co-signed years earlier so they could secure the house they wanted—but this was different. Illness changes the math in ways no one prepares for. He talked about applying for disability, and we gently explained how long the process could take and how hard it was to step back out of that system once inside it. There were conversations about tapping into retirement funds, choices that carried consequences he couldn't fully see through the fog of illness.

We tried to support him without overstepping, to offer guidance without taking control. It was a delicate balance—wanting to protect him, wanting him to feel capable, and knowing that chronic illness doesn't just drain the body. It drains savings, options, and the sense of safety you think you'll always have.

In the end, they made it through those months without our financial help, but the strain lingered. And when we later chose to pay for Greg's medical expenses with Dr. H, it wasn't because they asked. It was because we knew he would sacrifice his own care before risking anyone else's comfort. Maybe not at first, but as frustration grew, or if he didn't sense progress, we feared he might start skipping medications or cutting corners just to ease the financial pressure. That was the part that broke my heart the most.

There were moments when I sensed the strain between them, but I only ever saw it from a distance. And honestly, whose marriage wouldn't feel the pressure under circumstances like these? Chronic illness reshapes the emotional landscape of a home. Still, Greg never spoke poorly of Meagan; he was unfailingly loyal, always giving her the benefit of the doubt.

Once, after a difficult conversation, I texted him to say we would be there for him no matter what she decided. He didn't respond for hours. When he finally did, his message was simple: *"Mom, you misunderstood her. She's doing the best she can.*" His loyalty was unwavering—something I admired deeply, even when it left me wishing he didn't have to carry so much alone.

He didn't respond right away. The silence on the line carried everything he couldn't say—how worn down he was, how much he needed someone to believe him, how alone he felt inside a system that kept sending him home without answers.

Greg was at his breaking point, caught between pain, fear, and the quiet dismissal of doctors who couldn't see what he was living through. Each day without progress pushed him further into uncertainty.

Then his dad mentioned something—just a quiet possibility—but it stirred something in Greg. I heard it immediately, a new steadiness in his voice. The panic that had been gripping him loosened, replaced by something calmer. He wasn't waiting anymore. Something had changed in him, a spark of determination cutting through the fear.

He was going to chase the answer himself, no matter where it led.

CHAPTER SEVEN

The Descent

A couple of days later, on January 16th, Greg texted me after talking with his dad. Something in their conversation had pierced the fog he'd been trapped in—subtle, but unmistakable. The panic that had been spiraling all week paused just long enough for a single clear thought to surface.

By then, Al and I had thrown ourselves into the search for answers. We combed through articles, medical journals, and patient forums in every spare moment, looking for anything that might illuminate what was happening to our son. We compared notes constantly, passing every promising lead to Greg, hoping it might offer direction—or at the very least remind him he wasn't navigating this nightmare alone. And Al had stumbled onto something that would later prove closer to the truth than any of us realized.

Greg texted, "I think Dad is on the right track with Lyme disease—specifically Bartonella, which is a common co-infection. The problem is finding someone around here to investigate it. No one believes it's a real issue, and it's not something they see much of in med school. I've been trying to find specialized telemedicine options but have had little luck."

"Okay," I said. "Why won't your Primary Care Physician (PCP) at least run blood work?"

"I requested it today."

"Good. Keep on him until you get some answers. Doing nothing—just withholding testing—is not acceptable."

Throughout January, Greg buried himself in research on Bartonella. On the days he could manage it, he sat at his kitchen table with the lights dimmed and the screen brightness turned low, trying to spare his eyes. The house was quiet except for the soft breathing of Maple and Mona, the family dogs curled at his feet; their presence was the only steady thing in a world that no longer felt predictable.

He rubbed his temples as he read, pausing whenever the pain behind his eyes flared. Medical articles, case studies, and patient forums were spread across the table—tabs open, notes scribbled on a yellow legal pad, half-finished thoughts trailing off where the pain had forced him to stop. Then he'd rest his head in his hands, breathe through the ache, and try again.

Every time he brought his findings to his doctors, he hit a wall. They dismissed the connections he was seeing, and the more they brushed him off, the harder he dug. It felt like he was shouting into a void. Each visit ended the same way—no answers, no urgency, no one willing to look deeper. Meanwhile, his pain kept intensifying. He told me he was thinking about going to the Skagit County ER, forty minutes south of his home, because he didn't know what else to do.

Another week passed without a word from him, so I called.

"How'd the weekend go?" I asked. "Did you end up going to Skagit ER?"

"No," he said. "I'm trying to rest, but I might go this week. I just don't know what they'd do differently. They treat everyone the same, and they can't seem to think outside the box."

He hesitated before adding, "There's a naturopath in Bellingham I want to see. Maybe he'll believe me."

The following week, Greg scheduled appointments with both his PCP and the naturopath. I asked him what his plan was.

"Well, I don't think the PCP will even test me for Lyme, but the naturopath seemed enthusiastic when I talked to him on the phone."

"Please keep me informed. I also sent you some research articles that discussed intracranial hypertension—just something else to consider. Call me after your appointment if you can."

"I probably won't call, Mom, because I feel extra terrible today. I just want to get in bed, but I don't want to miss this appointment."

"Are you able to drive?"

"No, Meagan is driving me to town."

"Okay, thanks, Greg. We'll talk when you're able."

After meeting with the naturopathic doctor, Greg felt a cautious sense of hope and texted me a list of all the labs and tests the doctor planned to order. There were several, including a range of autoimmune panels. His heart lifted at the possibility of finally being heard as the last day of January approached. But that hope was short-lived.

On February 4th, Greg saw another ophthalmologist for a second opinion. He was told he did not have idiopathic intracranial hypertension, the condition originally considered when the MRI was done. IIH has all the symptoms Greg was experiencing—severe headaches, vision problems, tinnitus, and back pain.

This doctor spent time with him, listened to his concerns, and reviewed the MRI results without dismissing him or pretending to know more than he did. Because he didn't.

After the visit, the doctor prescribed lisinopril for high blood pressure. I asked Greg how his head was feeling. I hoped that if his blood pressure normalized, maybe the pain would ease. That was my prayer for him, anyway.

"Maybe a bit," he said—his answer felt less like certainty and more like an attempt to give me something hopeful to hold onto. He went quiet then, the kind of silence that comes when someone is trying hard not to unravel.

He hesitated, and when he finally spoke, the words came out in a tight rush.

"There's still something else wrong."

"Okay, Greg. Keep digging. You're getting closer."

I wasn't confident he was getting any closer, but I didn't want him to lose hope, so I said, "Well, that's another box checked off."

By mid-February, some of Greg's lab results came back. His Epstein–Barr antibody numbers were extremely high. When I mentioned this to friends who asked about his health, I often heard, "Oh, that's no big deal. I have EBV," or, "Everyone has EBV."

Ninety-five percent of the world's population carries Epstein–Barr, and for most people it lies dormant and causes no symptoms. Some young adults—myself included at twenty-one—develop mononucleosis from EBV. Those weeks are still a blur: drifting in and out of sleep, my body too heavy to lift from the mattress, the smallest effort leaving me trembling with exhaustion.

Even on the days I convinced myself I was well enough to work, my boss would take one look at me after a couple of hours and say, "Lynnette, go home. We've got you covered."

I could barely keep my eyes open long enough to eat, let alone function. It was the first time I understood what it meant for a virus to take over your life.

"So maybe he's got mono," I rationalized. "He's fatigued, sleeps a lot, and is in a great deal of pain."

EBV is an opportunistic virus that reactivates when the immune system weakens. If doctors couldn't identify or address whatever was affecting Greg, how could I expect anyone else to grasp what was happening? Most of my friends had met Greg during his many trips to Florida, so their questions came from a place of kindness, not judgment. Still, no one could truly understand what he was experiencing.

Throughout February, Greg spent most of his time sleeping, researching, and seeing doctors. Nothing improved. His pain was constant. Even though we were ready to come to Washington at his request, Greg asked us to wait until April.

"The weather will be better," he said. "And maybe I'll know something by then."

I sent Greg an article about a Yale study discussing EBV reactivation and symptoms similar to his. Researchers referred to it as post-vaccine syndrome, noting prolonged spike protein in blood serum as one of its markers. It was one of the research areas we were becoming familiar with. Greg responded:

"I read that too, and although it sounds similar, the study subjects showed symptoms 4–10 days post-vaccine. My symptoms appeared about

18 months after my last vaccination. Still could be, I guess. Thanks for sending it, Mom."

Greg was right about the timing—nothing in the literature explained symptoms appearing so long after vaccination. But as we learned from Dr. H later, the body doesn't always follow clean timelines. A dormant infection like Bartonella can simmer quietly for years, and sometimes the immune system only collapses after a final stressor. It didn't mean the vaccine *caused* anything; it simply meant that the sequence of events wasn't as straightforward as the studies suggested.

On February 20th, Greg saw the naturopath again. The doctor had given him a B12 injection at his previous visit, and Greg—grasping at anything that might help—asked for another one.

"I'm not sure if it helped, but it didn't have any negative side effects either."

The doctor planned to start him on supplements to support his immune system and wanted to treat the EBV, but he still didn't know what was causing Greg's head pain. For reasons Greg couldn't understand, the doctor still hadn't ordered tests for the other pathogens.

Greg believed it would help to address the inflammation in his body, so I offered what I could. I had been seeing a practitioner in Maine at The Center for Natural Healing and was taking supplements for pain and inflammation.

"I can send you some Cat's Claw and nettle tinctures if you think you'll use them, Greg."

"Okay, Mom, sure. I'll try anything at this point. I made nettle tea from all the plants in our yard."

There are plenty of nettle plants in Washington. We had a lighter moment reminiscing about when his father and I moved there from Maine, and I kept getting stung brushing against the plants in the backyard—three years before Greg was born.

"What the heck is this?" I had asked, my legs and hands numb and tingling.

A native Washingtonian laughed and told me the stingy nettles had "initiated" me. "Gotta watch out for those. They'll get you every time."

On March 3, 2025, a small earthquake rolled through Washington in the early morning hours. Greg slept through it, though the dogs startled awake, barking at the sudden tremor under their paws. When he heard about it later, he only shrugged. Most people barely felt the shake; Greg felt nothing at all.

The real aftershocks were inside him—sharp, unpredictable waves of pain that rippled through his body long after the earth had settled. While the world moved on from a tremor no one remembered, Greg was still bracing himself for the next jolt, the next surge, the next reminder that something deep within him was shifting in ways no one could explain.

A few days later, Greg had appointments with both his ophthalmologist and his neurologist. He saw the neurologist first—the specialist he'd waited more than two months to see. The doctor, compassionate and soft-spoken, well into his seventies, studied Greg with a kind of weary uncertainty. He guessed Greg had picked up a virus and said it would simply take time to heal. With no real answers to offer, he prescribed gabapentin for the pain.

"I liked him, Mom," Greg said afterward. "He seemed caring, just… unsure what's going on. I'll try the medication."

I nodded, though a knot tightened in my stomach. I had never found gabapentin helpful for pain. Still, this was his decision, and we would support him. What else could we do?

The ophthalmologist's appointment was worse. More of the same—another injection in his eye, another $400 bill, another six-week follow-up. Greg wouldn't have minded the cost if the injections were helping, but he felt himself slipping, not improving.

"I can't keep doing this," he said, his voice cracking at the edges. "Do you know how stressful it is to have a needle poked in your eye with no anesthesia?"

My heart ached for him. He was exhausted, the pain was relentless.

The doctor also discussed a surgery called a vitrectomy, which involves making tiny incisions in the eye, removing the vitreous gel, and replacing it with saline or silicone oil to help the retina heal. I didn't know much about it, so I ran it by my brother-in-law, Paul, an ophthalmologic research doctor in Dallas, TX. After I explained Greg's situation, Paul told me that most patients require cataract surgery within six to twelve months after a vitrectomy.

I passed that information on to Greg. He must have decided against it because he hasn't had the procedure.

Because of his limited vision, Greg could no longer drive safely. A retired friend of mine offered to take him anywhere in town or around the county. She didn't feel comfortable driving to Seattle—two hours away on a stressful highway—but Greg wasn't seeking care there anyway. He appreciated her availability, especially since Meagan was stretched thin with graduate school and work. So far, he had gotten to all his appointments without outside help.

In March, Greg added a mix of immune-support supplements to his routine—vitamins, herbs, probiotics—anything that might help his body fight back. He found that doctors couldn't grasp the severity of his pain and kept taking a "wait and see" approach to his suspected viral illness.

He wanted answers, and he didn't believe he had a virus—other than EBV—and without lab orders, he had no path to a diagnosis that explained why his world had collapsed.

At the end of March 2025, he showed his PCP the purplish marks on his skin and tried again to discuss testing for Bartonella. Instead, the doctor suggested testing for Cushing's disease, an autoimmune disorder. The test, the dexamethasone suppression test, involved taking a pill at night and having an early-morning blood draw.

Greg wasn't eager to do it. He didn't think the doctor was right. I encouraged him anyway.

"Just eliminate it from the list," I said. I asked about his eyes.

"Not great. I still have a lot of visual snow and floaters."

I changed the subject.

"How about your benefits and work? How much more time will they give you?"

"Not much. The doctor is filling out paperwork, and I need to check in with HR to see what they need. I've already been out for three months. I don't think they'll give me any more time."

Apparently, they didn't. His return-to-work date was April 1st. But his back was hurting, and he spent another week in bed, struggling to stand or walk. I suggested Epsom salt baths and gentle stretching—small things, but all I could offer.

The Cushing's test came back negative, as he expected. He returned to work on April 8th, and we arrived the next day. We didn't want to disrupt their home life, so we stayed in a travel trailer our friends had set up for us on their property in Ferndale.

Each day we drove fifteen miles to Greg's house to pick him up, then twenty-two miles to drop him at Nature's Path, repeating the pattern in reverse at the end of his shift. It was exhausting for him, and he didn't feel welcome back at his management job. Without a diagnosis to explain his absence, he had no answers for his coworkers or his boss—and, more painfully, no answers for himself.

We could see how sick he was. As his mom, I wanted to tell him everything would be okay, but I couldn't say that with any certainty. So instead, we focused on supporting him and spending as much time with him and his family as we could.

We arrived just before Easter, and Meagan invited us for brunch. I was grateful for the gesture; I knew she was stretched thin with work, graduate school, and caring for Murdoch, and it meant something that she wanted to share the holiday with us. She made a beautiful meal— quiche, fresh fruit, everything prepared with the same care she'd always brought to her cooking.

But beneath the surface, there was an unmistakable strain. I found myself unsure where to place my presence—whether to help in the kitchen or stay with Greg in the living room. The air felt delicate, as if everyone was trying their best but carrying more than they could comfortably hold. There was an awkwardness in the room that even the dogs sensed, making themselves invisible in the corner of the room. Greg made small attempts at humor that Meagan didn't respond to, but I could see she was doing what she could in a moment that offered no easy footing for any of us.

Al felt the tension immediately; he has never been one to pretend things are fine when they aren't. I tried to stay steady, to be gracious, to meet everyone where they were. Watching them together—two people who had loved each other since middle school, now navigating something neither of them knew how to fight—was quietly heartbreaking.

At home, the signs of how long he'd been sick were everywhere. The weather was beautiful, and we wanted to help Greg clean up his yard. He hadn't been able to keep up with it during the two years he'd been sick. The grass and weeds were over two feet high, and the tractor with the mower deck had been sitting idle. It needed troubleshooting before it would run again. It took a couple of days—some parts, some rewiring—but eventually the engine turned over. Completing that long-overdue task felt good, even if it underscored how much Greg had been unable to do.

It was heartbreaking to see so many of his projects unfinished. Greg has always had remarkable talents—woodworking, turning bowls on his lathe, pottery, mechanics, small engine repair, solving electrical problems most people would abandon. Their hundred-plus-year-old property held several outbuildings he once dreamed of restoring. Some were half-finished; others had slipped further into decay. Standing there, surrounded by the remnants of his creativity, it was painfully clear he no longer had the desire, energy, or strength to pursue the work that once defined him.

It was the first time we truly grasped how much of his life this illness had already stolen.

CHAPTER EIGHT

The Search for Answers

When his naturopath stopped returning calls, something in Greg finally broke. He told me the doctor had no secretary, handled all his own scheduling, and had gone on vacation without completing the lab work they'd discussed at his first appointment. One afternoon, after yet another unanswered voicemail, Greg pushed back from the kitchen table hard enough to make Maple and Mona lift their heads. He ran a hand through his hair, exhaled sharply, and muttered, "I'm done waiting."

He started searching for another doctor that same day. When his PCP still refused to order the tests he requested, Greg drove straight to the lab in frustration and asked whether he could order the Bartonella blood work himself. They told him he could pay for the antibody test out of pocket for $150, but it came with significant limitations. A negative result didn't rule out the disease; the test simply wasn't sensitive enough to detect such a covert pathogen.

That's exactly what he got. The test was negative, but it didn't deter him.

"I'll just look into better testing or a more complex panel," he said. "I'll also have to find a doctor who will work with me."

"Those results are not unexpected, Greg. Just see it as another completed step on your journey."

In his spare time, even as his eyes burned and blurred without relief, Greg kept researching. It was one of the few things that made him feel like he still had some control. Near the end of April, he emailed me an article about the relationship between EBV reactivation and long Covid.

"I found it very interesting that the EBV testing and positive results I had aligned with the author's assertions."

The article was ninety-three pages long, dense and technical, so he highlighted the parts he wanted me to focus on.

I could tell Greg was getting closer to something. His texts had taken on a different tone—faster, sharper, as if his mind was racing ahead of his body. He'd been piecing together studies, charts, and medical theories with a kind of intensity that reminded me of him as a child, when he'd take apart a toy just to understand how it worked. Only this time, the stakes were unimaginably higher.

Then one afternoon my phone rang. His name lit up the screen, and before I even answered, I felt it—something had shifted. There was an urgency in the timing, the kind that comes when a person finally sees a pattern that's been hiding in plain sight.

"Mom," he said the moment I picked up, "I think I finally understand what's happening."

I could hear papers rustling, the familiar rhythm of him pacing while he talked. He didn't pause long enough for me to respond.

"I've been going back through everything," he said, "and when I put it all together, the other inference is that long Covid presents as a cellular illness, not a respiratory one. It's a compelling argument for long Covid from the vaccinations I received, but no doctor has considered testing me for the spike protein because I don't even know if I ever had the virus."

What I understood him to be saying was that long Covid might not behave like the initial infection at all. It could hide in the cells, lingering in ways that didn't show up on standard tests. And for Greg, that possibility wasn't just scientific—it was personal. It was a way to make sense of the chaos inside his body. A way to believe he wasn't imagining the pain. A way to feel less alone.

He took a breath, then said it plainly, as if naming it might give him something solid to hold on to.

"I think I have long Covid—plus EBV reactivation, and maybe Bartonella. It's the only thing that explains all of this."

Then he moved into the language he'd taught himself in the sleepless months of trying to decode his own symptoms.

"My research into endothelitis and micro-thrombosis—both cellular conditions— shows they're often precursors for diabetic retinopathy."

The words came fast, dense, as if he were trying to outrun the fear behind them. I didn't understand the terminology the way he did, but I could hear what it meant for him. "Endothelitis" wasn't just a term; it was the burning tightness in his legs that made walking feel like wading through fire. "Micro-thrombosis" wasn't an abstract concept; it was the needling pressure behind his eyes that blurred the edges of the world.

What he was really telling me was that his body felt like a map of things going wrong, and he was trying—desperately—to find the legend that made it all make sense.

This kid definitely inherited his father's brain for advanced science and microbiology. I had taken the basics—anatomy and physiology—but nothing like this. Whenever he used terms I didn't recognize, I'd ask him to spell them so I could look them up later. He never hesitated. He assumed I could learn the language too, and in his own way, that was a kind of faith.

And yet beneath all the terminology, I could feel the fear he didn't say outright: *If these conditions are connected, maybe there's a reason my vision is failing. Maybe someone should have caught this. Maybe I'm running out of time.*

He continued, his voice tight with urgency.

"I'd already done my research regarding mitochondrial activation and ACE2 inhibition, which is why I started taking methylene blue."

He said it as if these were ordinary concepts, as if every parent should understand the biochemical pathways their child was trying to untangle. I'd ask him to repeat unfamiliar terminology so I could look it up later—not because I doubted myself, but because I wanted to stay inside the world he was fighting to understand.

I tried to imagine what "mitochondrial activation" felt like to him—not a theory, but a sensation. The way his muscles trembled after standing for only a minute, as if every cell were revving too hard and still not producing enough power to hold him upright. And "ACE2 inhibition" wasn't just a mechanism; it was the suffocating heaviness in his chest when he tried to breathe deeply, the feeling that something essential inside him had been switched off.

After we hung up, I sat with everything he'd said. Then I immediately texted him back, encouraged that he was seeing the bigger picture—but also aware of the truth he didn't say aloud: he was terrified. His mind had always been the sharpest tool he had, and lately he'd confessed that even that felt like it was slipping.

I knew enough from other people's stories to understand why that scared him so much—how infections like Bartonella could masquerade as schizophrenia or dementia, and how sometimes, by the time anyone realized what it really was, the damage couldn't be undone. He was trying to save himself with the only tools he had left—his mind, his research, and the hope that somewhere in all the science, there was an answer that could give him his life back.

"I give you a lot of credit for doing all the research and making educated guesses about which protocols to follow. Dad is reading the article, and we can all discuss it together when he's done. We love you very much and support your journey wherever it takes you."

When I hit send, the room felt unbearably quiet. I stared at my phone, wishing I could reach through it and take even a fraction of his fear into my own body. I wanted to protect him, to fix this, to be the mother who always knew what to do. And part of what made that fear so heavy was knowing what he'd been forced to do on his own.

Greg knew he wouldn't be able to get the prescription medications he believed he needed. He explored ways to obtain antibiotics from countries with fewer restrictions than the United States. Canada was only a thirty-minute drive, but their regulations were similar to ours. Ordering online from India felt too risky, and although medications were available in Mexico, he would have had to travel there—something he was far too ill to do.

So, he turned to self-treatment: ivermectin from the farm store and methylene blue purchased online.

I was with him the day we went to buy the ivermectin. Greg was actually happy that day— genuinely happy. After years of being the one to travel to Florida to see us, he finally had us in Washington with him. Al hadn't been back in seven years, and I'd only returned once in five. Just having us there seemed to lift something in him.

Before we even stepped inside the store, he and his father were already outside admiring the tractors, slipping easily into their old rhythm of comparing horsepower and attachments. I didn't know then that the tractor we'd left him—the beautiful green John Deere Al had been so proud to pass down—had fallen into disrepair during the years when illness had drained his strength. He didn't tell us, but I could sense it in the way he looked at the new tractors: hopeful, a little guilty, as if buying a new one might be easier than admitting how much the old one had suffered right alongside him.

Inside the store, the smell of hay wrapped around us—normally a scent I loved—but that day it made my stomach tighten. Rows of rubber boots lined the wall, the kind meant for people who spent their days mucking stalls. Greg moved past them with purpose, still buoyed by the excitement of having us there, and headed straight for the livestock medications.

When he found the ivermectin, he picked it up with a confidence that startled me. I took the box from him and read the label carefully. It was unmistakably for horses.

"How are you going to know how much is okay to take?" I asked.

He didn't hesitate. "I can calculate it by weight," he said, as if it were a simple equation. He actually took the first dose in front of me. He squeezed the paste onto his finger, hesitated for half a second, then put it in his mouth.

My stomach dropped. I knew he was desperate, and I understood why he was willing to try anything—but watching him swallow something meant for a thousand-pound animal terrified me. What if he miscalculated? What if this made everything worse? I didn't say it out loud, but the fear sat heavy in my chest.

"Yuck, this is awful," he said, grimacing.

My heart dropped. I wasn't sure it was safe—not at all—but I also knew there was no convincing him otherwise. He was a man on a mission, willing to do anything to feel better. The paste was apple flavored, but clearly only in theory. I tried to lighten the moment—"Only a horse could appreciate apple-flavored medicine"—but even I could hear the strain in my voice.

And beneath that strain was something older, something I hadn't thought about in years: the memory of Greg at ten years old, newly diagnosed with diabetes, standing in our kitchen with a bravery I didn't yet have. I had been terrified—afraid his life would depend on my vigilance, afraid I would never be able to keep him safe. But he looked up at me with steady eyes and said, "Mom, I can do this."

And he meant it. Within days he was insisting on giving his own injections, quietly lifting his shirt in the classroom or stepping into the restroom if the teacher preferred. He didn't hide it or act embarrassed. He explained what he was doing to the other kids, teaching them why it mattered, turning something frightening into something ordinary. He wasn't afraid then. He was confident, certain, already stepping into a strength I hadn't realized he possessed. And he proved himself right. He managed his diabetes with a maturity far beyond his years, showing me—again and again—that he could carry what life handed him.

Now, watching him choke down that apple-flavored paste, I felt the same ache I'd felt back then: the desperate wish to protect him, paired with the painful knowledge that he was the one stepping forward with courage. He was still fighting. Still trying to save himself. Still saying, in his own way, *I can do this.*

We knew about the ivermectin because we were standing right beside him when he bought it, but we didn't understand the full extent of what he'd been doing on his own until we settled into Washington in April. I had reservations, of course, but desperate times require desperate measures. What frightened me most was the possibility that his despair might push him toward even more dangerous choices if he continued treating himself without medical guidance—or if he ended up with tainted medication from overseas.

I didn't fully understand the condition he believed he was addressing, but I understood the feeling of abandonment. He felt dismissed by his healthcare providers and unsupported by a medical system that seemed unwilling—or unable—to investigate his unexplained illness any further.

Under normal circumstances, I would never advocate for self-treatment—certainly not for something this mysterious, this uncertain, this frightening. If you have a cold, fine: take some cough syrup, make chicken soup, rest.

But whatever Greg had, it wasn't a cold. There were no simple remedies, no over-the-counter fixes, no clear path to follow. There were no real answers for self-treatment at all. And yet I couldn't stop him from taking matters into his own hands. He had done his homework, and he was desperate for relief.

It reminded me of the true story of the parents who searched for a cure for their son's devastating nerve disease, adrenoleukodystrophy (ALD), after doctors gave them little hope for his survival. Refusing to accept that prognosis, they developed a mixture of two cooking oils that slowed the progression of the disease and kept their son, Lorenzo, alive until age thirty. Most children with ALD succumb within two years of diagnosis; he lived twenty-four years beyond his.

Their journey was portrayed in the 1992 film *Lorenzo's Oil.*

In April, Greg still hadn't found a doctor willing to work with him. We kept suggesting he contact Mayo Clinic or Cleveland Clinic, where they would run comprehensive diagnostic testing until they found an answer. But the idea of getting on an airplane with the level of head pain he was experiencing was unbearable. He felt trapped—confined to his local community and the limited medical care available to him.

His father and I dove headfirst into research on Bartonella, EBV, Covid-19, long Covid, and studies on vaccine-related complications sometimes referred to as post-vaccine syndrome. I was determined to learn everything I could because his life mattered, and research was one of the few tangible ways we could help him.

Driven by the desire to help Greg, I immersed myself in medical literature and discussed findings with the family. The shared effort expanded our knowledge and deepened our resolve to support him in every way possible.

As a family, we kept exchanging articles, studies, and insights—anything that might help us understand what was happening to him. Every new piece of information fueled our determination. Research became the one thing we could do, the one place where we felt we weren't powerless.

My lifelong love of learning resurfaced with a force I hadn't felt in years. In high school, I'd been honored as the "most studious student," a small recognition that now felt strangely relevant. In those days, I was always chasing A's, refusing to settle for anything less than a perfect score. But now, none of that mattered. I was in uncharted territory, with no syllabus, no outline, no clear path to follow. For the first time in my life, it felt like I wasn't making the grade. We couldn't find the answers because there were too many questions.

By the end of April, one truth had become painfully clear: Greg was fighting this battle largely on his own. The medical system had failed him, and he was doing everything in his power to save himself. All we could do was stand beside him, learn as much as we could, and hope that somewhere in the growing stack of research, an answer was waiting to be found.

CHAPTER NINE

Forward Momentum

Between January and May 2025, something in Greg began to shift. At the start of the year, every phone call carried the same heaviness. Sometimes he answered with a flat "Hey, Mom," the kind of greeting that told me more than anything he said afterward. Other times there was a long pause before he spoke, as if he were gathering the strength just to begin. He sounded worn down by symptoms that refused to budge and terrified by the possibility that they never would. Each day seemed to confirm his worst fears, and the lack of answers left him feeling helpless.

His frustration deepened with every medical appointment. He came to see the doctors he met as incompetent or indifferent—unable or unwilling to help him understand what was happening. More than once he said, in a voice edged with exhaustion, "They don't care. They just want me out of the office." His anger wasn't really about them. It was about the fear underneath—the fear that no one would ever figure out what was happening to him.

He rejected the idea that his condition was psychological. He also dismissed the possibility that his nightly drinking—the one thing that gave him a few hours of escape—might be making things worse. I understood why he clung to it. When your world is falling apart, you hold on to whatever numbs the edges. But I also knew we couldn't ignore it forever.

Before we talked to him about next steps, I made a list of everything he had already done in search of answers. He had quit smoking two years earlier, a habit he'd picked up in culinary school—common in that high-pressure world—but giving it up hadn't improved how he felt.

"Quitting was supposed to help," he told me, his voice tight. "But I'm just getting worse."

We began by acknowledging the progress he had made before gently outlining what needed to happen next. His responsibility was clear: he had to stop drinking. His father and I explained why this mattered and how we would support him.

As expected, he pushed back.

"There's only so much doctors can do for you, even with a diagnosis. The rest is up to you."

"I can't sleep at all."

"Have you tried melatonin or even CBD?" I asked. "A lot of people use it for sleep now."

"I already take melatonin. I guess I could go to the dispensary and ask for something for sleep."

It was a hard conversation—one I had dreaded—but Greg relented.

"Okay," he said quietly. "I know you're right."

It felt as though he just needed to say it out loud. He quit drinking that day.

Still, I worried about relapse—especially when Meagan and Murdoch were gone for the weekend. During those times, I checked in more often. He always said he was doing fine, and I wanted to believe him, but those weekends alone had to be hard.

Recently, I asked how that part of his recovery was going. It had been a year since he'd stopped drinking.

"Well, honestly, I kind of wanted a cold beer a couple of weeks ago when we went to the Nooksack Brewery for pizza," he admitted. "Beer was never my thing, but I tried one."

He paused before continuing.

"I didn't like it and didn't finish it. I can honestly say I don't have cravings anymore."

"That's a good thing, Greg. You don't need more stress in your life right now."

By May, even though his physical health hadn't improved, Greg continued to take intentional steps toward caring for himself. He approached his healing like a research project, testing ideas methodically—almost like a scientist working through a hypothesis. Something in him had steadied—not physically, but internally. There was a quiet determination that hadn't been there before.

Along with the medicinals he was already using, he added new strategies. He adopted a keto diet, made rest a priority, and explored saunas and other natural healing practices. His symptoms persisted, but these efforts showed his commitment to taking control of his health and doing everything in his power to move toward recovery.

He was also closing in on finding a physician who understood his condition—someone who could offer a clear diagnosis and create a treatment plan to support his healing. All the groundwork he had laid, the research he had done, and his willingness to embrace self-care seemed to be aligning. The saying often attributed to Buddha came to mind: *When the student is ready, the teacher appears.*

That thought felt especially fitting when Greg texted me on May 27.

"Have you ever heard of fascial Counterstrain?" he asked. "I found a new ILADS-certified doctor who just moved to Bellingham, and I've scheduled an appointment for next week. It's worth seeing what she says, or whether she recommends additional testing."

"No, but it sounds promising. I read her bio—she might be the doctor you've been looking for."

I'll admit I had to look up what ILADS meant. The International Lyme and Associated Diseases Society is the leading medical society devoted to treating Lyme and associated diseases.

The timing felt serendipitous. Dr. H had just moved to Bellingham and was opening her own practice. A naturopathic physician, she treated vector-borne illnesses and other complex conditions. She had also battled chronic Lyme, Bartonella, and mold-related illness herself.

Despite how sick Greg was, the internal work he had done seemed to prepare him for this moment. He was ready for the next stage of his journey: naming the illness, understanding it, and working collaboratively to address it.

The following week, on June 6, he met Dr. H in her new office in Fairhaven, a historic district of Bellingham. The space was nothing like a typical medical clinic—soft light instead of harsh fluorescents, old brick walls that held their own history, and the quiet click of Juni's paws on the floor as she greeted him at the door, Dr. H's therapy dog in training.

"Great visit. She drew blood and ordered labs." "We met for a full hour. I haven't had more than 15 minutes with a doctor in over two years."

For the first time, he felt heard. Dr. H agreed to test for conditions that previous physicians had dismissed as unlikely or unnecessary.

Hallelujah, I thought—finally, someone who was listening.

Her lab orders were extensive. When Greg told us the cost of the testing, I felt that familiar tightening in my chest—the fear that money might become yet another barrier between him and the answers he needed. We offered to cover everything related to testing and treatment. At that point, nothing mattered more than giving him a chance to move forward.

The initial testing for Bartonella and related infections totaled around $1,500. Insurance covered only some of the standard labs. Only two laboratories in the United States processed Bartonella testing, and Greg was told to expect a three-week turnaround. Supplements would also be out of pocket, classified as "alternative medicine." Every new detail made the situation feel heavier, but I kept reminding myself to stay steady for Greg. He needed hope, not my panic. But the truth was, it wasn't calm at all. It was a mix of panic and a strange, fragile excitement.

Within days, he received results from a local lab for his SARS-CoV-2 antibody and spike protein testing. Greg's result—1391.0 U/mL— was shockingly high. For a moment, I just stared at it, unable to reconcile the tiny "<0.8" of the normal range with the number in front of me. I felt a cold rush of fear, followed by the familiar need to steady myself before calling him. It was another piece of the puzzle, but it didn't bring clarity. Only more questions.

Three years after the Covid vaccination, his body still seemed unable to clear the spike protein—something I had read was being reported in a subset of patients with persistent immune dysfunction. Most people, the literature said, cleared it within days or weeks. But Greg wasn't "most people," and that truth pressed harder on me with every study I opened.

I kept reading, trying to make sense of what was happening inside him. Study after study described immune responses that echoed pieces of Greg's experience—neurological inflammation, disruptions to protective barriers, retinal complications. None of it offered answers, only more questions. And none of it felt abstract. It was my son.

Greg rarely voiced his fear, but we felt it nonetheless: that his doctors would never identify the cause of his eye damage before his vision was gone.

For two years, he underwent treatment without improvement or reassurance. Each appointment ended the same way:

"We'll wait another six weeks and see if there's improvement."

And each time, there wasn't.

With every new procedure and injection, there was a renewed sense of hope that the progression could be halted. Yet despite mounting disappointment, Greg held on to the belief that there was another diagnosis—one that could explain all of his symptoms and offer a viable path forward.

Despite his persistence and optimism, the answers he sought remained elusive, leaving him and those around him grappling with uncertainty and concern for his future.

Greg's excitement grew around the three-week mark, when he expected the Bartonella results to come in. He checked the patient portal every morning, sometimes more than once, hoping for a message from the lab or from Dr. H. Each time he found nothing, he tried to shrug it off, but I could hear the strain in the way he said, "Still no update."

Week four came and went. Still nothing.

"Give them a couple more days, Greg," I said, trying to keep my voice steady from three thousand miles away. I didn't want him to hear the fear rising in me.

Week five arrived, and the silence felt heavier.

"Greg, maybe you should call Dr. H," I said, doing my best to hide the panic creeping into every word.

He didn't argue. He didn't sound angry or frustrated. Instead, he went quiet in that way he sometimes did—the kind of quiet that wasn't calm at all, but a way of bracing himself. When he finally spoke, his voice was steady, almost too steady.

"I'll wait a little longer, Mom. It's fine."

But it wasn't fine. Not for him, and not for me. His calm felt like something he had chosen—a thin shield against the fear that no one would ever figure out what was happening to him. Beneath that quiet resignation, I could feel it: something was deeply wrong, and we were no closer to understanding what it was.

The doctor had said three weeks. At five weeks, he still knew nothing. Every day of silence tightened the knot in my chest. We were still standing in the dark, waiting for someone to turn on a light that never came.

Greg had no answers. And the silence only grew louder as the light grew dimmer.

CHAPTER TEN

Diagnosed

Six weeks passed before Greg finally called the lab to find out why he still hadn't heard from Dr. H or received his test results. After all that waiting in the dark, the answer was almost absurd: the lab had mixed them up and assumed they'd already been delivered.

On July 22, the day before his follow-up appointment, he accessed the paperwork online. When he texted me, I sensed a heaviness in his words—discouragement, maybe even resignation.

"I got the lab results from Dr. H. She had to pester them to send them again. I emailed you a copy. The way I see it, there's not much there. Looks like there was something in the past, but there are no strong positives. It's interesting to read though, and I'll be meeting with her tomorrow morning."

I tried to keep my response simple, steady.

"Okay, Greg. Now you can focus on what you need to move forward. Let us know what she comes up with."

He called the next day after seeing Dr. H. Even with all the research he'd done, he couldn't interpret the lab results the way she could. Nor could I. They were just a jumble of numbers and difficult medical terms. I could hear the effort in his voice—the way he was trying to explain something complicated while still processing it himself.

"I was right," he said. "They only tested a few types of Bartonella, so they couldn't tell which one I have. But she said it doesn't matter—she wants to start treatment *now*."

He paused, as if gathering the next piece.

"She said more testing would just waste time and money. I emailed you everything she gave me."

I opened the email while we talked. The diagnoses were listed plainly:

Bartonella. Epstein–Barr virus. Covid Spike Abs. Low VEGF.

I already knew what the first three were, but what was Low VEGF, I asked?

"That means I'm not getting enough blood flow to my nerves, so there's not enough oxygen."

"Oh," I said. "What do you do for that?"

"Do you see all the supplements on the second page?" He asked. "Those should help, Mom."

I felt a brief sense of relief as I read through the treatment plan. He had finally received a diagnosis for the disease he suspected he had back in January—but it was now the end of July. Greg's suffering had gone on far too long because so many doctors were unfamiliar with, or unwilling to investigate, anything outside the narrow boundaries of their training. *I hope it's not too late.*

For months, he had been self-treating with supplements and herbal protocols—a result of his own careful research and our persistent search for answers. But what he really needed were the antibiotics he couldn't get without a prescription, and the medical guidance to target the exact pathogen he was fighting. With Dr. H, he finally had both.

Dr. H explained the science of Bartonella to him—how the bacteria can hide inside red blood cells, how it can suppress the immune system, how it can linger for years undetected. She told him that in a healthy person, the immune system often keeps it under control. But Greg's immune system had been weakened by years of Type 1 diabetes and the reactivation of Epstein–Barr virus.

After his appointment, Greg called again, trying to simplify her explanation so I could understand.

"Basically," he said, "this thing hides in your blood cells and messes with your immune system so it can keep spreading. That's why it's so hard to get rid of."

"Okay," I said. "I think I understand that."

"She thinks I've had this for years," he added quietly. "Way before Covid."

"Well, we know you've been sick for over three years."

"No," he said. "She thinks I've had Bartonella way longer than that. It just came to life *during* Covid."

"Oh, wow. That's crazy, Greg."

As he talked, Murdoch's diabetes diagnosis came back into focus. At the time, none of us connected it to anything beyond genetics and bad luck. But now, after everything we had learned, I asked whether he had ever wondered about the timing of Murdoch's diagnosis and his Covid vaccine.

"Yes, Mom," he said. "It's crossed our minds."

It wasn't an answer—just a window into the uncertainty we were all living with. Greg's Bartonella diagnosis illuminated more than his own suffering; it cast a long shadow across our family's medical history, raising possibilities I wasn't yet ready to confront.

He went on to explain that many people never know they've had Bartonella. Some show no symptoms at all. Others experience only mild discomfort. Often the body recovers on its own.

"Remember that Yale article we read about post-vaccine syndrome?" he asked.

"Yes, but you didn't seem to fit the criteria. Their symptoms appeared within days, and yours didn't surface for months."

"I know," he said. "That's why it never made sense to me. But it keeps popping up."

"Well," I said, "it looks like you're a unique case study."

He gave a tired laugh—the kind that held both relief and exhaustion.

I read through Dr. H's report slowly, letting each line settle. Eight new medications—some prescriptions, others supplements—layered on top of what Greg was already taking. An individualized treatment plan, specific to his symptoms and his immune system. It was more than a protocol; it was a roadmap for a body that had been fighting in the dark for years.

Because Bartonella is a bacterial infection, Greg would eventually need prolonged antibiotic treatment. But Dr. H didn't start there. Her first priority was strengthening his immune system so he could tolerate the harsher medications later. It made sense, but it also meant the road ahead would be long.

There were two full pages of instructions: when to take each pill, which ones required food, which ones didn't, what to do if he reacted badly. She warned him about herxing—a flu-like reaction that happens when the body begins killing off bacteria faster than it can clear the toxins. I remembered seeing the term before, but I had to look it up again. It sounded miserable, but it was also a sign that treatment was working.

She also prescribed a very clean diet: no sugar, no gluten, no alcohol. Half a plate of vegetables at every meal. Berries every day. Grass-fed or wild meat or fish. It was strict, but Greg didn't complain. He had already lived through years of feeling sick; discipline wasn't the hard part. The hard part was the waiting—the not knowing if any of this would help.

He still needed to document his symptoms daily, but he had already been doing that for months. He had a system. Greg always had a system. The pills, drops, and tinctures all had to be taken at specific times, and he created a spreadsheet to keep track of everything. He sent me a picture of the pink Trader Joe's lunchbox he bought to carry his daytime supplements and medications to and from work. It was so full the sides bulged.

"Wow," I said. "That's insane."

"Well, it helps me stay organized," he said. There was a hint of pride in his voice—the kind that comes from finally having a plan.

"She also told me to be prepared to feel a lot worse before I see any improvement."

"That's tough," I said, "but at least you know what to expect. I'm sure it's a relief to have answers now and to start a treatment program targeted at your specific symptoms. With everything she's suggesting, you're facing a full-time job."

"Yeah," he said. "But it'll be worth it just to feel good again."

Greg felt a deep sense of gratitude for meeting Dr. H, even with the unease of what lay ahead. With Juni, her therapy dog, Dr. H approached her patients with a kind of steady, grounded compassion that Greg hadn't found anywhere else. The two of them were going to get to know each other well—and make a strong team.

Greg was ready to move forward with unwavering determination, intent on eliminating the infection that had quietly taken root in his body for years. His sense of anticipation and hope spread to those around him, inspiring confidence that he could overcome the illness.

What he didn't yet understand was the magnitude of the fight ahead. The setbacks. The side effects. The days when progress would feel impossible. The moments when hope would flicker and nearly go out.

But he didn't need to understand all of that yet.

At that moment—standing at the threshold of a diagnosis he had waited years to receive—Greg's optimism carried him. And for the first time in a long time, it carried me too.

The path forward was difficult, but it was finally visible. And that was enough.

CHAPTER ELEVEN

The Hostile Takeover

Something in Greg's voice told me the illness wasn't finished with him.

Greg wanted to believe he was finally on the right path. Dr. H had warned him that treatment would make everything worse before it got better, but for the first time in months, he felt supported and seen. After fighting this unnamed disease alone for so long, he was ready to begin the battle as part of a team. With Dr. H beside him, he believed they could finally confront the pathogen that had been tormenting him for years.

We all hoped improvement would follow. But none of us understood how ruthless the illness would become once treatment began.

In those early weeks, Greg and I talked frequently. Now that we finally had a name for the illness, my research had direction instead of desperation.

"I've been reading more about how you get Bartonella, Greg."

Even though he probably knew as much about it as any specialist, he listened while I tried to make sense of what I'd learned.

"What'd you find out, Mom?"

"Well… it can come from so many places. Wild animals, pets… even the ones we've had around the house. And cats carry it the most. Flea bites, scratches—anything that breaks the skin." As I spoke, my mind kept drifting back to Smokey, the cat we rescued when Greg was sixteen, and all the dogs that were part of our home. Then to the years after he married, when he was surrounded by even more animals—his own dogs, the two old cats he adopted, and all the creatures he cared for on the property. Any of them could have been the start of this.

He let me talk, the way you let someone work through a fear you've already made peace with.

"Where do you think it came from?" I asked.

"Not sure yet, Mom. But Dr. H and I have discussed some theories."

Pinpointing the exact source was nearly impossible. But as I wrote this memoir, stirring up memories I hadn't touched in years, one moment rose to the surface: the time Smokey tangled with that raccoon in the woods when he was around three.

The infection that followed was deep and stubborn, and I spent nearly ten months tending to that cat, cleaning the wound, giving antibiotics, trying to keep him alive. Greg probably wouldn't even remember it now. But I do. And as these old memories resurface, I find myself wondering—not with certainty, just with possibility—whether something might have been passed along in that fight, carried quietly afterward in the cat we all loved so much.

Another memory followed close behind: those strange purple lesions Greg developed in his late teens and early 20s. By then, Smokey had been part of our family for years—always curled up beside Greg, brushing against his legs, leaving tiny scratches that seemed harmless at the time. Had something been carried quietly through those years, slipping into Greg's bloodstream long before any of us understood what it meant?

The truth is impossible to pinpoint. But writing this story has shown me how many forgotten moments might have shaped the path we're walking now—how many possibilities were woven into our lives without us ever realizing it.

For so long, Greg had only mentioned the marks on his skin in passing, and they went unnoticed by others. In hindsight, those lesions were significant. As a healthy young adult, his immune system may have kept the infection suppressed, allowing it to remain dormant or minimally invasive.

It wasn't until two years ago, during a visit to Florida, that they came sharply back into view. We were at a local water park with Murdoch, and as Greg stepped out of the pool, dark purple lines streaked across his midsection—stark against the wet sheen of his skin, the water sliding off him in rivulets that made the marks look even deeper, almost bruised.

"How long have you had those marks, Greg?"

"Since my late teens. They've always been there."

"That's rather odd."

Murdoch tugged at us, begging for another ride, and the moment slipped away. But the image didn't. Those lines stayed with me—bold, unmistakable, nothing like the stretch marks I'd once assumed they were. Another clue tucked quietly into the past, waiting for its meaning to surface.

Looking back on Greg's medical history, doctors often attributed his symptoms to diabetes, especially fluctuations in blood sugar. He'd been hospitalized several times for severe hyperglycemia that required emergency care. That pattern continued in recent years, with ophthalmologists insisting his eye problems were diabetic retinopathy.

"They just don't want to consider that it could be anything other than my diabetes."

"What is Dr. H's perspective?"

"She doesn't want to commit to either theory, but she's treating the entire illness anyway. If my eyes get better, there's a good chance this infection is contributing to the damage."

With hindsight, I couldn't help wondering whether the intruder had been attempting its takeover during those earlier years—quietly advancing and weakening him while we remained oblivious.

As his immune defenses faltered, the once-silent invader began to advance. It settled into his eyes, causing internal bleeding, dark spots, floaters, and sudden drops in vision.

"I can feel it when it's happening, Mom. I have little time before the spots block my vision."

One afternoon, he called while driving home from work in a blinding rainstorm. The moment I answered, I could hear the storm through the phone—rain slamming the windshield, the wipers struggling to keep up.

"Oh no…" The panic in his voice tightened something deep in my chest.

"What's going on, Greg?"

"It's happening, Mom. The spots are coming in fast. I've got to get home before I can't see anything."

I gripped the phone so hard my fingers ached, trying to steady my voice even as fear surged through me.

"How close are you?"

"Not far. I'm in town—almost home."

The rain hammered harder, a steady roar swallowing the sound of his engine. Then suddenly—nothing. Just silence.

"Greg?" My breath caught. "Greg, are you home?"

A beat. Then finally: "Yes. I'm in the driveway. I'm just going to wait a few minutes before I go inside. This is so frustrating… the spots are still there."

"I'm so sorry, Greg." My voice felt small, useless against the storm pounding on his car and the one happening inside his eyes.

There was nothing I could do except stay with him, holding space across three thousand miles.

"I'm going in now, Mom. Talk to you soon."

"I love you, Greg."

"Thanks, Mom. Love you too."

When the call ended, the despair hit me all at once. I felt completely helpless, gutted by the truth that I couldn't protect him, couldn't stop what was happening inside his body. The weight of that helplessness was almost unbearable, and the tears came the way they often did in those days—quietly, slipping down my face where no one could see. Al stayed steady, practical, grounded in his way. I carried the emotional truth on my sleeve.

Besides the eye damage, Greg lived with a rotating storm of pain and neurological symptoms—headaches that flattened him, cognitive fog that stole his clarity, and the kind of traveling pain Meagan described as "every day it's somewhere else in his body."

I immersed myself in research on Bartonella, Lyme, and other vector-borne diseases. These illnesses are on the rise worldwide, often misunderstood and difficult to diagnose. Many patients go untreated for years.

One clinician told me that people who don't recover from Lyme often have an undetected Bartonella coinfection. Its victims live with suboptimal health for years.

As I dug deeper, I found studies suggesting Bartonella could contribute to psychiatric symptoms. Some patients who didn't respond to standard medications improved only after receiving antibiotics. The pattern was hard to ignore.

A doctor misdiagnosed me with depression years earlier. I took the medication, went to therapy, did everything I was told—and nothing changed. It wasn't until someone finally checked my thyroid that the real problem came into focus.

That experience stayed with me. It taught me that when someone isn't getting better, the solution isn't always more treatment—sometimes it's a different question.

As a mental health therapist for thirty years, I often encouraged clients to talk with their physicians to rule out underlying medical issues. So when Greg's personality began to shift—when the irritability and heaviness settled in—it was hard not to see it through that same lens. Something deeper was happening to him. Knowing what Bartonella could do, it was impossible not to wonder whether it was part of the picture. One afternoon, I finally asked him the question that had been circling in my mind.

"Greg… why do so many doctors dismiss all of this? Lyme, Bartonella, the co-infections. Why won't they even look at it?"

He sighed, and I could hear the weariness in it. "Mom… I don't know. I really don't. I think half of them just don't want to deal with something this complicated."

"But why not at least consider it?" I asked.

"Because they've seen too many weird claims," he said. "And then when someone like me walks in with real symptoms, they lump us all together. It's easier for them to shut down than sort through it."

He paused, and when he spoke again, his voice was tighter.

"I've had so many appointments where I can tell the doctor's already made up their mind before I even finish a sentence. They don't want to hear what I've figured out. They don't want to talk about possibilities. They just… shut the door."

I could hear the frustration rising in him—the same frustration he'd felt when a doctor pushed him toward a diagnosis he knew didn't fit.

"And honestly," he added quietly, "I'm tired. To get help with something like this, you need a doctor who's willing to stick with you for the long haul. Months. Years. And most of them just… aren't."

His words stayed with me long after the call ended. They explained so much—not just the medical controversy, but the silence he kept running into, the doors that kept closing. And they made the shifts in his personality even harder to ignore.

I was beginning to understand something I hadn't grasped before. The weight in his voice, the sharp edges of anger that didn't sound like him— they felt less like moods and more like something pushing its way forward. Some researchers even referred to this pattern as "Bartonella rage." And even from three thousand miles away, I felt my whole body stiffen when that tone slipped through—the one he tried so hard to hide.

Greg already had a diagnosis, but the emotional shifts during those long waiting weeks became impossible to overlook. It was as if the illness had its hands on him, tightening its grip in ways I was only just beginning to recognize. Watching that happen from across the country was its own kind of heartbreak, and all I could do was wait for answers that refused to come.

Greg had been trying for months to make sense of the strange lesions spreading across his torso—red streaks that seemed to appear out of nowhere. When he finally showed them to his doctor, hoping for answers, the appointment ended almost as quickly as it began.

"It looks like Cushing's," the doctor said, barely glancing at the marks before turning back to his computer. Greg tried to explain why he thought it might be something else, something he'd been researching on his own, but the doctor didn't want to discuss other possibilities. "Let's rule out Cushing's first."

When the test came back negative, Greg expected the conversation to open. Instead, the doctor dismissed the lesions entirely. "Then it's nothing to worry about."

Greg told me later how stunned he felt—how quickly the door had closed, how little space there had been for questions. It wasn't the first time he'd been brushed aside, and it wouldn't be the last.

As I dug deeper into Bartonella and the other vector-borne infections that kept appearing in my research, I began to understand why Greg's illness had been so hard to identify. These diseases live in a strange no-man's-land of medicine—too complex for simple explanations, too inconsistent for standard testing, and too unfamiliar for many physicians to feel confident diagnosing.

They don't behave the way infections are "supposed" to behave. They hide, they shift, they mimic other conditions, and they slip through the cracks of the very systems meant to detect them.

The more I learned, the more I realized Greg had found himself in the middle of a medical controversy he never asked to be part of. Bartonella, Lyme, Babesia—often called "stealth pathogens"—can burrow deep into tissues and cells, evading the tests doctors rely on.

A person can be sick and still test negative. And when the labs come back clean, the burden of proof shifts onto the patient. Symptoms get dismissed as stress, anxiety, diabetes, or "just life." I saw that happen to Greg over and over again.

I saw how many people were living in that same limbo—sick, searching, unheard. Some specialists insisted Bartonella could cause neurological and psychiatric symptoms; others dismissed the idea entirely. Some believed it could lie dormant for years; others argued it couldn't.

The disagreements weren't just academic. They shaped the care people received, the treatments they were denied, and the years they lost trying to prove their own suffering.

For Greg, that controversy wasn't theoretical. It was personal. It was the reason he spent years fighting an invisible enemy with no name—the reason his symptoms were blamed on diabetes, or stress, or "just getting older." He had to become his own researcher, his own advocate, his own detective.

As I read more, an unsettling truth began to take shape: Greg wasn't an outlier. He was part of a much larger pattern—one medicine is still struggling to understand. These illnesses don't just infiltrate the body. They seep into the spaces between specialties, into the gaps between lab results and lived experience, between what doctors are taught and what patients endure.

That gap—that silence—was where Greg had been forced to live for years. As the weeks passed, it became painfully clear that he was no longer battling a quiet, hidden illness but an aggressive force intent on taking more of him each day. I could hear it in his voice, see it in the way his symptoms shifted and multiplied, feel it in the helplessness that settled between our phone calls.

Bartonella was no longer lurking in the background; it was tightening its grip with a violence none of us had anticipated. Yet even as the illness pressed harder, Greg held on to a thread of determination—a belief that the right treatment might finally slow the descent.

As frightening as those days were, that small, steady hope became the bridge that carried us into the next phase of his journey—one defined not by recovery, but by the first real steps toward fighting back.

CHAPTER TWELVE

Laying The Foundation

With a proper diagnosis at last, Greg began the first real steps of treatment in early August 2025. Those first two months were intense. He followed a strict regimen of supplements, antivirals, antimicrobials, and support for neuroinflammation. Some were meant to quiet the inflammation that had been raging through his body, others to steady his nervous system or help blood flow more easily to his brain. There were treatments aimed at strengthening his immune system, and others directed at the long Covid, EBV, and Bartonella that had taken such a toll on him.

As he stepped into this demanding regimen, I found myself holding a complicated mix of emotions. My heart felt full and relieved, and sad all at once. We all know we can't live our kids' lives for them, but that doesn't stop our hearts from breaking when they're hurting. Watching him step into this next phase—hopeful, exhausted, determined—was its own kind of ache.

In those early weeks, I tried to find small ways to stay connected to him, even from across the country. All we could do was support him from afar, and I tried to tell him often how much he meant to me. One afternoon, I sent him a text— one of those messages that comes straight from the heart.

"Greg, I can hear how hard this has been for you, and I'm really proud of how you keep pushing through, even on the days that feel impossible. You've always had this quiet strength, and it shows in the way you keep showing up for yourself. We're right here with you through all of it. And I love you."

He wrote back, "Thanks, Mom."

Even his short replies felt like small signs of life returning—tiny reminders that he knew he wasn't facing this alone. It was enough. We were simply grateful he had finally found someone who believed him—someone willing to explore the complexity of his illness instead of dismissing it. Dr. H treated him with the kind of respect every patient deserves but doesn't always receive, even from the people closest to them.

But even with a doctor who finally understood him, the emotional toll of the past years still clung to him. By then, Greg's illness had progressed to a place where he felt isolated in his suffering. People didn't believe him, or they lacked compassion, or they assumed he just needed psychotherapy.

He was angry—an anger that was painful and frightening to witness—and I began to understand what some researchers meant when they described "Bartonella rage." Bartonella—often known in its simplest form as "Cat Scratch Disease," though Greg's illness was far more complex than that—was reshaping him in ways that were heartbreaking to witness. He was no longer the calm, tender-hearted, gentle man he had always been.

As both his mother and a psychotherapist, I found myself trying to understand the roots of this anger while also respecting the limits of what therapy could offer him in that moment. I usually advocate for counseling, but when someone is living with intense pain, vision loss, and cognitive impairment, the last thing they want is to talk about their problems only to have them dismissed as psychological. Greg's scientific mind needed clarity first. He needed to feel well enough to think, to make sense of what was happening to him. He needed answers. And he had been to therapy as a teenager, so he understood how it worked.

"Don't get me wrong, Mom," he said one day, "but I think therapy right now would be a joke."

"I get it, Greg. You want to understand what's happening to your body, not to talk about your feelings. Just stay focused on the treatment program Dr. H designed for you. Pay attention to how you feel with each new drug or supplement. Keep doing the saunas, the acupuncture, the gentle stretches, and massage. Keep up with your journal."

"I'm doing the best I can, Mom."

"That's good enough, Greg."

These conversations reminded me how limited we were by distance. His father and I were his biggest allies, but being three thousand miles away made it nearly impossible to help with the daily nuances of his life. We did everything we could to keep the lifeline strong, offering support while trying not to intrude on the independence he'd carved out for himself years earlier.

It was important to us not to take that independence from him. Our role often felt like walking a tightrope—balancing between being present and stepping back, making sure he knew we were there while still honoring the boundaries he needed to make his own decisions.

His independence had always been a point of pride, but the medical system had eroded his trust. By then, he'd lost count of how many physicians he'd seen over the past couple of years. The system had worn him down, and he'd developed a hardened edge toward it. In his mind, if a doctor didn't know what they were looking at, they should say so—and send the patient to someone willing to explore the mystery instead of pretending it didn't exist.

When a patient finally feels heard and receives a plan for treatment, there's a kind of exhale that happens—a release of tension they've been carrying for far too long. That moment of being believed can be the first real step toward healing.

As the weeks went on, Greg continued exploring different therapies. In early September, he met with Dr. H for Counterstrain Therapy, a gentle manual technique designed to release tension in the body's connective tissue. After the session, he sent me a quick update.

"Pretty interesting appointment. The touch is light, but I definitely feel like things moved around inside my head."

Later that day, Greg forwarded me a YouTube link about Bartonella. "This is the best description I've heard of how I've felt for the last eighteen months. It's a good listen."

For the first time, he felt someone was speaking his language. I watched it immediately. Hearing someone else articulate what he'd been living through made my chest tighten—relief that he finally felt understood, and grief that it took a stranger's video to do it. I texted him back, wanting him to feel supported.

"That is a great video. I like the approach you're taking with Dr. H—treating the disease with an individualized plan, because what works for one person may not work for another. See yourself as the healer you are, using multiple tools and resources. It will be the most challenging yet rewarding journey your life takes you through."

"You have a solid start now, and you know the hills you'll have to climb and the valleys you'll pass through. Just remember who you are along the way, regardless of what others think. You know we always have your back and support your journey forward, even if it sometimes feels like two steps forward, one step back. Thanks for sending this. I'll share it with Dad."

He wrote back, "Thanks, Mom. I thought it was great and did a good job of describing how I get overwhelmed at minor things."

For a brief moment, it felt like we were finding a rhythm—small exchanges that reminded me he was still fighting, still paying attention to the shifts inside himself. But a couple of weeks later, everything shifted.

"I met with the pharmacist at the endocrinologist's office today, and my A1C is 5.7."

For a moment, everything inside me lifted. After months of setbacks and discouragement, here was something solid—a number that meant his body was finally responding. For Greg, it was more than a lab result. It was hope.

"Wow," I wrote back. "That's great."

A 5.7 might sound ordinary to most people, but for someone living with Type 1 diabetes, it was astonishing—a sign that something in his system was finally cooperating.

And then, as if hope could arrive in layers, he added one more piece of news. "Oh, Dr. H prescribed ketotifen for me to start at night. Sounds like an interesting drug. I should have that early next week, since a compounding pharmacy has to make it for me."

"That's great, Greg. I'll look that one up. I've never heard of it before."

Ketotifen wasn't just another medication; it was another tool, something meant to quiet the inflammation that had been tormenting him for so long. Another possibility. Another small step forward.

But healing rarely moves in a straight line. The week wasn't all good news. Greg had another eye bleed—something that always caused him a great deal of anguish. He said he could feel it happening: first a shift, then the sudden loss of central vision, leaving him with only a narrow ring of peripheral sight. Black spots and floaters would cloud his vision for weeks as the blood slowly dissipated. He told me it set him back about three months, and the discouragement in his voice was unmistakable.

And then, in the midst of all this, life kept moving. A few days later, it was his forty-second birthday. I wrote to him:

"Happy Birthday. Embrace all the love that surrounds you on this day. Your birth was the *best day of my life*, filling me with the most profound and unforgettable love imaginable, and I am forever grateful for you. I know you've faced tough challenges, but your persistence in healing will bring you substantial rewards someday. LOVE you bunches."

His typical response came back: "Thanks, Mom."

I could feel the heaviness behind those two words—the way discouragement had begun to settle over him again.

"Greg, believe in the power to think yourself healthy. Our minds are powerful. Use yours wisely."

Another soft reply. "Thanks, Mom."

He was always grateful, even when I wasn't sure he believed a word I said. Still, I hoped that somewhere beneath the exhaustion and frustration, he held on to the idea that healing was possible—that the tools, the medicine, the support, and the love surrounding him could help carry him forward. He had to know how deeply we loved him. It was all we had to give. The rest was up to him.

As he stepped into the next phase of treatment, the reality of what lay ahead began to settle in. The weight of it pressed in—he would need every ounce of strength he had. We didn't know it then, but the progress would come in inches—slow, uneven, and often invisible to him.

Greg struggled to see any change at all, caught between pain and impatience, convinced he was standing still.

Our role shifted too. Our job became noticing what he couldn't: the tiny shifts, the quiet improvements, the moments when something, anything, was just a little better than the day before. We held those small victories up to him like lanterns, hoping they would help him keep moving forward when the path felt impossibly dark.

And even then, we had no idea what was coming. We didn't know it yet, but the hardest part of his treatment was still ahead.

Looking back, I can see how fragile that moment was—how much we were holding without realizing it. We were clinging to hope in its smallest forms, trusting that each faint glimmer meant something, even when the road ahead was hidden from us. At the time, all we could do was love him through the uncertainty, not knowing how much deeper the journey would take us.

CHAPTER THIRTEEN

The Turning Point

As September drew to a close, I sensed a quiet readiness in Greg—a small but unmistakable shift, as if he were finally standing at the edge of the next phase. He was eager to move into what he called the "meat" of his treatment program.

"Mom, I have another Counterstrain appointment today," he said. "And I think I'm going to ask her if I can start antibiotics now. I'm ready."

Greg had taken very few antibiotics in his life. Aside from his diabetes, he'd always been healthy, the kind of kid who bounced back from everything. But Bartonella was different. I'd learned enough by then to understand that this illness didn't play by simple rules. It had no rules at all.

He'd been thinking about this for weeks, trying to understand the mechanics of what was happening inside him. He explained it to me once over the phone, his voice carrying that mix of frustration and fascination he lived with now. "It's like the bacteria hide," he said. "They build these little shields so the meds can't get to them."

He meant the biofilms and the fibrin layers—words I never expected to use in everyday conversation. The idea that something microscopic could build a fortress inside his body was both surreal and terrifying. Some clinicians use enzymes to help break down those barriers before introducing antibiotics. Greg already knew this. He'd been taking enzymes on his own for months, convinced they were helping his body reach what had been walled off.

He'd also done his homework on the antibiotics themselves—what combinations were used, why one medication alone often wasn't enough, and how different drugs targeted different stages of the bacteria's life cycle. He wanted to understand the logic behind every step. It made him feel less like a patient and more like a partner in his own recovery.

Dr. H had walked him through all of it. She reassured him that when the time was right, they would choose the combination together. She also warned him that treatment wasn't a sprint. It could take months—sometimes years—depending on how deeply the illness had settled in.

She explained pulsing too, the start-and-stop rhythm some people use. The breaks can sometimes draw the bacteria out of their hiding places, making treatment more effective when it resumes. And the pauses give the body a chance to breathe, which Greg desperately needed after two years of feeling like his system was constantly under siege.

By the time his appointment came around, he was ready for answers. After his appointment, Greg texted me.

"Hi, Mom."

"Hi, Greg. How'd the Counterstrain go?"

"Man, that feels great."

"Oh, that's wonderful. It's good to hear you say that. I hope it lasts a while."

"Yes, I hope so too. I think she got some stuff draining into my head today."

"Must be a weird feeling," I said.

"Yes, it is weird. But to be fair, everything has felt weird for the last two years."

Then, almost casually, he added, "I am going to start some antibiotics just to see."

My heart jumped—hope, worry, relief, all tangled together. "Is she concerned about the antibiotics? What did she prescribe?"

"Azithromycin and Cipro, maybe? Not sure yet. You need two to start, but she didn't want to prescribe the rifampin yet, which is what I wanted, but it is very harsh."

"Yes, it is, Greg. Just be mindful of your gut health at the same time."

He already knew that. He knew more than most adults would ever want to know. But saying it made me feel like I was doing something— anything—to help.

Greg's understanding of his condition impressed Dr. H, but he was eager to move faster than she felt his body could manage. He was going to have to follow the pace she set, even if every part of him wanted to sprint.

On the last day of September—National Sons Day—I texted him.

"Happy National Sons Day. Although I don't know why we need a specific day to say I love you, when I feel that every day for you. I am sad that you've got yet another eye bleed, and I wish I could take it all away. Love you always."

A moment later, his reply appeared on my screen—the same two words he always used, but this time they felt warm, almost gentle.

"Thanks, Mom."

My heart swelled. I just love that man-boy so much.

Even in his discouragement, he met me with gratitude. I held on to that—held on to him—to the quiet hope that love could reach across the miles and steady him when nothing else could. The rest was his path to walk, no matter how much I wished I could walk it for him.

I didn't know what the coming months would bring, but one thing was clear: Greg was still fighting, still reaching for the light, and we would be right there beside him in every way we could. A foundation was forming—quietly, imperfectly, but unmistakably. Something in him was beginning to shift, even if he couldn't feel it yet.

At the time, I didn't think much beyond the relief of forward motion. Only later did I realize how much the antibiotics would shake things up— first in ways I couldn't see from afar, then in ways none of us could ignore. It became a turning point, though at the time I believed it was simply the next hopeful step forward.

There were days ahead when Greg couldn't see any sign of progress at all. But even in the chaos, tiny shifts appeared—faint and fragile, visible only from the outside. We saw the light long before he could, and we held on to it for him until he could see it himself.

We didn't know it yet, but the hardest stretch was still ahead of him.

CHAPTER FOURTEEN

The Breaking Point

On October 14, 2025, I flew from Maine to Florida, where we would spend the next seven months in our retirement community. Once we let people know we'd arrived and settled in, Greg and I texted, and I asked the proverbial question.

"How are you doing?"

"Okay. I'm so tired at work. All the energy I regain during the weekend is gone pretty quickly. Otherwise, all good."

"Yeah, that sucks. Didn't Dr. H suggest you might have to take more time off when symptoms got intense?"

"Yes, but I don't want to. I have to keep trying."

"Okay, Greg. Hang in there."

Even through text, I could feel the strain in him — the way he was pushing himself past what his body could reasonably manage. The following week, Dr. H suggested he add a new probiotic to his regimen. He was already feeling miserable, and just as she warned him, the next few days were rough.

Being so far away made everything harder. When Greg hit those moments of overwhelm, he pulled inward, shutting out the people around him. His wife could hear the shift in his tone before he said a word—the clipped answers, the agitation under the surface—and she would call me, her voice tight with worry.

I slipped into that strange blend of therapist and mother, a role I never wanted but knew how to hold. I called him every few hours, listening for the tremor in his voice, the edge that told me he was barely holding on. He never hung up on me, even when he was flooded. And I never reacted to the intensity I heard. I stayed steady, naming what I could, letting the rest move through him like weather.

That role wasn't new to me. I had been in it years earlier, when Greg and Meagan were teenagers and then young adults, sitting together in my therapy office to talk through whatever they were struggling with. I was grateful they trusted me, even as I worried about the complications of being both the mom and the therapist. They told me things I sometimes wished I didn't know, but they trusted their "stuff" was safe with me. They don't come to me together anymore—life has changed—but in moments like these, the old dynamic resurfaced. Greg still reached for the steadiness he had always known I could offer.

And now, the stakes were higher. What some researchers describe as Bartonella-related emotional dysregulation was no longer an abstract concept. The depersonalization he'd questioned months earlier was now unfolding in real time, and I could hear it in the way he spoke—like he was standing just outside himself, watching emotions he couldn't quite control.

One afternoon, during one of those difficult stretches, I asked gently, "Greg, have you eaten anything today?"

"No," he said, flat and distant.

He was alone—Meagan and Murdoch had left hours earlier to stay with her parents—and the thought of him sitting in that house with nothing grounding him made my chest tighten.

"Okay," I said. "I want you to go into the kitchen and find something to eat. Anything. I'm going to call you back in thirty minutes."

When I did, the shift was unmistakable. The old Greg was there again, sitting at the table eating a grilled cheese sandwich. His voice was calmer, softer around the edges. He sounded wrung out, but present. Himself.

Once the storm eased, he always came back to me like that—tired, drained, but anchored again. He was honest when I asked about the depth of what he was experiencing. He told me that everything I had gently inquired about—the intrusive thoughts, the surges of anger, the dread—was real for him.

He tried to protect me from the worst of it, but even the fragments he shared were enough to reveal the truth. And beneath those slivers was a fear he couldn't disguise—a fear of thoughts that didn't feel like his own.

I knew he wasn't telling me everything, but even the part he allowed me to see made my chest tighten. Everything I had learned—stories, case reports, accounts from others I'd only read about—made it clear how profoundly Bartonella could affect a person's mind. The emotional turmoil, the distorted thoughts, the sense of slipping away from oneself… it was all too real.

It's terrifying to imagine someone you love going through that. Even more terrifying for the person living inside it, unsure whether it's safe to speak the truth out loud. When his filters dimmed and the intensity surged, he poured everything into me, and I held it—not just for a while, but in the way a mother does, unable to set down the weight of her child's suffering.

This illness wasn't just physical anymore; it was eroding the edges of who he was. It was mentally and emotionally draining for Greg, and for all of us who loved him. In those weeks, it felt as though he was standing at the very edge of himself, and all we could do was hold steady and pray he wouldn't slip any farther.

CHAPTER FIFTEEN

The Spark Returns

"Dr. H told me this would happen," he said one day, his voice small but steadier than it had been. The intensity of the previous weeks had eased just enough for him to name what he was feeling instead of being swept away by it. It wasn't recovery, not yet, but it was a shift—a softening at the edges, a hint that something inside him was beginning to settle.

"We know, Greg. The most important thing is not acting on thoughts that don't feel like your own and finding someone safe to talk to when things feel overwhelming. Dad and I are always here. Any time of day or night, we can talk through whatever's happening. You won't always feel this way."

By the time he finally replied, "Thanks, Mom," his voice had steadied.

Every time he came back to me like that, it was a small gift—a sign that the worst had passed for now. And in those quiet moments afterward, I always found myself searching for something I could offer him, some thread of comfort or perspective he might hold on to. Most days, the inadequacy pressed in, grasping for words that might ease even a fraction of what he was carrying.

Watching him struggle made me think about how hard he'd pushed himself for so many years, how much weight he'd carried without ever slowing down. Young people are always chasing their dreams, trying to get ahead, climbing the corporate ladder. We did the same thing when we were young—it's what everyone around us expected. Only now, with a little age and perspective, did I see how that constant push can make you miss the things that actually matter.

One evening, as I watched the sun sink behind the trees, I wished Greg could feel even a moment of the peace I felt. I sent him what was in my heart:

"Life isn't supposed to be nonstop stress. Let the sunset remind you that you're here to live, not just grind. You need moments of wonder and rest—not as a reward, but because they matter."

He replied quickly:

"Thanks, Mom. Yes, a good reminder."

I could almost hear a small exhale in those words—a tiny softening that told me he'd let the thought land.

When discouragement crept into his messages, I reached for whatever steadiness I could offer. I wanted him to remember something I had learned the hard way—that peace mattered more than proving anything. So I texted him:

"Your peace matters more than proving anything. It's okay to say no. Boundaries aren't selfish—they're healthy. When everything feels heavy, shrink your world to what you can actually handle and breathe."

His response came after a longer pause: "Thanks, Mom."

It felt quieter, almost tired, but still grateful. Even when he didn't have much energy, he reached for those two words. His world had already narrowed, and he was slowly learning what he could release. It was one of the few ways he could protect himself when everything felt like too much.

When his mind was foggy and decisions felt impossible, I reminded him of something I'd told countless clients over the years—advice I now found myself offering my own son:

"Slow down. Breathe. Let your heart guide you when your head feels scrambled."

And then, the same thing I tell anyone going through a major life upheaval:

"Don't make any big decisions until all this is behind you."

"I know, Mom. I won't," he wrote back. His voice—even through text—sounded steadier then, like he'd found a little footing again. And I held on to that.

As his mind steadied, the practical pieces of treatment came back into focus. Later that day, he told me he'd had his blood drawn. He'd been asking Dr. H about starting rifampin, and she needed a baseline before deciding whether it was the right next step.

Some doctors use rifampin alongside other medications when treating severe or persistent bacterial infections. Greg never mentioned anything about neuroretinitis, but the more I learned about his eyes, the more I wondered whether his vision problems were caused not only by diabetic retinopathy but also, at least in part, by the Bartonella. Or maybe it was just a mother's intuition trying to make sense of what didn't add up.

A couple of things nudged me toward that conclusion. First, the retinal hemorrhaging began only after Covid, right when all his other health issues erupted at once. Second, the many ophthalmic treatments he'd endured over those two years hadn't stopped—or even slowed—the bleeding. And now, as of this writing, Greg told me his eyes were better than they'd been in a long time.

"I don't want to jinx it by saying that," he said, "but maybe the antibiotics are working."

In my heart, I whispered a quick prayer that he was right. Maybe the beast inside him was finally growing weary. Maybe the new medicine would mount its own quiet offensive, loosening the grip of the organism that had stolen so much from him.

In my mind, I pictured the rifampin going after the bacterial cells, each one wrapped in the little biofilm coats they'd built to protect themselves. The enzymes had already weakened those coats, and I imagined the antibiotic slipping through the cracks to do its work.

If only it were that simple. They're tricky little bugs—intent on settling into their host, creating a cozy home for themselves while slowly wearing down the body they inhabit.

But creativity and imagination have their place in facing chronic illness. Sometimes the only way to stay afloat is to hold on to images of healing, to lean into hope rather than fear. Positive energy doesn't cure disease, but it can steady the mind and soften the edges of suffering. Fear, anger, and negativity can drain what little strength a person has left.

Watching Greg fight made me think about the role hope plays in healing. We all know people who have beaten the odds against cancer or other chronic conditions, often because they believed in their ability to recover and could picture themselves living a healthy life again. That kind of inner vision doesn't replace treatment, but it can be a powerful companion to it.

Hope isn't abstract to me; I've seen what happens when it's present—and when it's gone.

In contrast, some individuals lose hope under the weight of their suffering and slip away when they no longer have the will to keep fighting. That was the case with my mother, who contracted the superbug MRSA after a failed colon resection in the summer of 2007.

Her doctor told me she was experiencing what they called "failure to thrive," turning away from food and water. She grew weaker and passed away two months after her surgery. It was a painful reminder that no matter how much we want someone to stay with us, they must also want to live. Mom was exhausted and disheartened, and all my attempts to lift her spirits or encourage her recovery simply couldn't reach her.

Thinking about her made me even more aware of how fiercely Greg was still fighting. A few days after his blood draw, he received the results, and everything looked good. Greg could start the medication as soon as it arrived from the pharmacy. Dr. H planned to check his liver function every three to four weeks.

I reached out to him on Veterans Day to see how he was doing and whether he planned to start the medication.

"I started rifampin last night," he said. "It hit me pretty hard, but in a good way. Lots of muscle spasms, butterflies, but no pain or nausea. It seems to reduce my head pressure even more. Fingers crossed, but I think it is doing something substantial."

"GOOD NEWS. Thanks for letting us know. It sounds like something good is happening. So glad to hear, Greg."

Four days later, I checked in again.

"Hi Greg. Have you been tolerating the rifampin for the last few days?"

"Going okay. Pretty rough on the stomach. There is a lot of nausea, so the thought of eating makes me sick, but I'm hanging in there. I still think it's helping my head symptoms."

I told him I'd read that taking probiotics a few hours after rifampin might help with stomach issues. As usual, he was already ahead of me.

"Yes," he said. "I'm taking two different probiotics about three hours after my morning dose."

Greg had another Counterstrain therapy appointment on November 20th. I asked him to let us know how it went and what Dr. H had said.

"I'm feeling better this week in terms of nausea and appetite, so I seem to be getting used to the meds. My back is still bothering me in the morning. Counterstrain should feel good today."

A moment later, another text came through.

"I spent some of my work fitness money and ordered a balance board to try regaining some of my core strength and balance."

"That's great, Greg. Whatever keeps you focused forward is good. It was wonderful hearing you talk about your hopes and dreams the other day—you never know, they really can manifest if we believe in the possibility."

I added, "Dream as big as you want. Bastyr, (the naturopathic university in Seattle) doesn't have to be a pipe dream. We believe you have what it takes to reach something like that. Keep putting your dream out there, and the universe will meet you if that's the path you're meant to take. Love you, and I hope you feel better after the Counterstrain."

A few days earlier, we'd had a two-hour phone conversation—the first time in years he had sounded like his old self. He talked about going back to college, about Bastyr in Seattle, about becoming a doctor—not a clinician, but a researcher dedicated to finding better treatments for vector-borne illnesses.

"The tuition's only two hundred thousand dollars, Mom," he joked.

"And with my science degree, I'm only one class shy of being able to apply to medical school. I think I could get it done before I'm fifty."

They were lofty goals, and I didn't know whether he truly intended to pursue them. But that wasn't the point. What mattered was hearing him dream again—hearing capability and confidence return to his voice after so long.

Maybe this abysmal time in his life would lead him toward something more purposeful. He had always imagined himself working in research and development in the food industry, but life had taken him in a different direction, and so far, he's spent his entire career in quality assurance. Like his father, he was brilliant in the sciences, and like me, he loved research and learning. Maybe a medical degree really was in his future.

I called him the next morning.

"How did you feel after your appointment yesterday?"

"Oh, pretty great. Unfortunately, the pain is back this morning. I think it is helping, though. One weird thing is that I'm waking up hungry. You know, I've never been hungry in the morning. As long as my labs stay normal, Dr. H is hoping I can do at least six months on the rifampin."

Later that week, we had another remarkable phone call—over an hour long. We talked about the simple pleasures in life, sharing moments that were lighthearted and genuinely uplifting. Greg's voice carried a hopefulness I hadn't heard in a long time. The conversation was different from so many before it—no talk of pain, no cataloging of symptoms or medications. Instead, it was easy and encouraging, full of possibility and positivity, a glimpse of the Greg I had been missing for years.

The next day, Greg texted to say he had messaged Dr. H and asked for a titration plan to help him taper off the gabapentin. He wasn't seeing a neurologist anymore and had decided he didn't need the medication long-term. Tapering off would at least reduce his daily regimen by six pills.

"Okay, good," I told him. "With all the other medications you're taking, I think it would be okay to stop the gabapentin."

Then I added, "By the way, it was so great to hear you laugh and joke yesterday. Something must be working."

"Agreed," he wrote back. "Something is working. Feel like there is a long way to go but also realizing I felt horrible for a very long time and just thought it was normal."

"Yes," I said. "We can look back and see it too. There will be a long and winding road ahead, but now you have a plan and a program to follow. You don't have to keep seeking diagnoses. It will be an interesting journey, seeing how your mind and body can change and heal. You will be a much better version of yourself overall."

"I hope so, Mom. I've been in survival mode for so long."

"We know you've felt horrible. It's human nature to convince yourself it's normal—or blame your diabetes, or your eating, or even drinking to cope. Just keep putting one foot in front of the other and follow the path that's laid out for you. It must be getting clearer up ahead. At least now you know what you're up against."

Let him dream—the bigger, the better. After everything he had endured, hearing possibility return to his voice felt like a gift. For the first time in years, he wasn't speaking from fear or survival mode, but from a place of hope. It simply felt good to hear that spark in him again.

CHAPTER SIXTEEN

The Long Road

His initial optimism faded as neuropathy and restless leg symptoms resurfaced soon after stopping the gabapentin. The spark was still there, but it flickered under the weight of returning pain. Healing, I was learning, wasn't a straight line. It was a long road—one that asked for patience, resilience, and more grace than any of us felt we had.

On December 10th, torrential rain hammered western Washington, warm enough to melt the mountain snowpack and send it rushing downhill. Greg had been at work earlier that day, and he told me later how the storm sounded inside the car on his drive home—rain pounding the roof so hard it drowned out the radio, wipers scraping at full speed and still losing the battle. The air inside grew damp and cold, carrying the smell of wet upholstery and mud from his shoes.

As the Nooksack River spilled over its banks, the surrounding landscape blurred into a sheet of moving water. Roads shut down one after another—Sumas, Ferndale, Everson—each closure forcing him to turn around and try another route. He said the tires hissed through standing water, the steering wheel vibrating under his hands as he navigated stretches that felt more like shallow streams than roads.

He eventually made it home, shaken but safe. When he stepped out of the car, he looked out over the raspberry fields below his house—fields that usually stretched out in neat rows—and saw nothing but water.

"Mom, I've got waterfront property now," he texted, sending photos that made my stomach drop. His house sat on a hill, but everything beneath it had disappeared under a muddy, rippling lake.

"I just feel like crap. I need to rest," he said when he called.

His voice carried a heaviness I hadn't heard recently—exhaustion layered with the kind of stress that settles deep in the body.

"Sounds like a good plan, Greg. That's the best thing you can do for yourself right now. Take as much time as you need." I kept my voice even, but inside something tightened. Every time he dipped after a stretch of hope, it pulled at a place in me I rarely let him see. I wanted to steady him, not add to the weight he was already carrying.

The floodwater took days to recede, but the weight of it—the weather, the symptoms returning, the sheer effort of navigating daily life—had already settled on him. Rest wasn't just deserved; it was necessary. And despite everything, a quiet relief settled in knowing he was finally giving himself permission to stop.

As Greg stepped back to rest, a sense of acceptance settled in too. This was where he needed to be—gathering strength, honoring his limits, letting the world slow down for a while. Healing asks for patience, and so does love.

I didn't know it then, but while Greg rested, something else was making its way toward me—a small, unexpected gesture he'd created long before this storm. It would meet me at just the right moment, carrying more meaning than either of us could have imagined.

CHAPTER SEVENTEEN

The Echo of an Old Gift

On Christmas Eve, an overdue package arrived from the Blaine post office, the kind of small, ordinary box that doesn't look like it could hold anything important. But Greg had told me to watch for it, and something in his voice made me pay attention. When I opened it and lifted out the wooden bowl, a quiet recognition moved through me—the sense that this wasn't just a gift, but a thread pulled from some deeper place. I didn't yet understand what it would unravel or restore. I only knew it carried a story that had been waiting for me to be ready.

For a moment I let myself imagine that Greg had made it recently—that his hands, steady for just long enough, had shaped this gift in the present. But when I turned it over and saw his initials beside the year '19, a different understanding settled in. This wasn't something new. It was something he had carried with him, something he chose to send back to me now, as if offering a piece of the past that had been waiting for its moment to speak.

And as I held Greg's bowl in my hands, that past began to stir—something soft, familiar, almost like a whisper from a place I hadn't visited in years. The smooth birch, the careful burn marks, the way the lid fit just so… it all carried a tenderness that felt older than the gift itself. And as I traced the carved initials on the bottom, a memory rose up, unbidden, from a corner of my life I had nearly forgotten.

And with that memory came another—a bowl of my own, tucked away for years, carrying a story I hadn't touched in a long time. A few weeks earlier, I had found a paper mâché bowl I made long ago, hidden in the back of a closet. It was bright and wild and covered in the story of my life—painted words spiraling around the outside perimeter, pictures pasted inside like tiny windows into who I once was. I called it my Memory Bowl. You had to turn the bowl to read it, just as I had once turned myself toward the world with bright colors and confidence.

I sat on the floor and read the words I had written as a young woman, and I cried. I had forgotten how vivid I once was. How much I loved hot pink and faux leopard print and crazy hats. How alive I was before my father died.

Before my mother's fear pressed itself onto me like a rulebook for survival.

I can still see the moment it happened. On the morning of my dad's funeral, everyone was waiting in the living room while I got dressed. I came out wearing the prettiest dress I owned—a hot pink polyester sailor dress with a pleated skirt and a wide flared tie. I had pulled on matching fishnet stockings, brushed my hair, and bounded toward the living room where everyone else stood ready. I wasn't a girly girl, not really, but I wanted to show my dad—thirteen years old and trying so hard—that I was going to be okay, that I could still find something bright in the middle of all that darkness.

The look on my mother's face stopped me cold. Then came her voice, sharp and breaking all at once. "Go take that dress off. We are not going to a party," she choked through her tears.

I was heartbroken, but I turned around and hurried back to my room, slipping into something quieter, something safer. Something that wouldn't make anyone look at me. I never wore that dress again; it hung in my closet after that, meant only for my eyes. Sometimes I would glance at it and run my fingers along the perfect pleats, holding the wide pink tie in my hands as if touching it might bring back the girl who chose it.

And then one day it was gone—a remnant of my past that disappeared without explanation—but the memory never left me. That was the day something in me went quiet. The brightness I'd felt just moments before collapsed in on itself, and as I walked back to my room, something in me pulled shut like a door.

But there was another part of the story I had forgotten—something I wrote in a moment of clarity I was too young, or too overwhelmed, to fully understand. I wrote about a presence, a soft white light that visited me through my teens in my basement bedroom, whispering that I was safe, that life would get better, that I would have to work hard and wait. And then, in words I barely recognized as my own, I wrote about an ally who would one day return the color to my life.

I wrote those lines at a time when Greg was becoming unmistakably himself—bright, spirited, full of color—and I loved watching that unfold. I didn't yet understand why it thrilled me, only that something in his wildness felt familiar, like a part of me I had set aside. When I made that bowl all those years ago, I must have sensed something I couldn't yet name. I must have known, somewhere inside me, that Greg reminded me of the girl I once was, the one who loved color and wasn't afraid to be seen.

And now, all these years later, he had sent me a bowl he made when his own life was full of possibility. A bowl he kept on a shelf, a piece of himself he chose to give back to me. An echo of an old gift, arriving at the exact moment I had rediscovered my own.

As I held Greg's bowl, the two memories—his and mine—seemed to speak to each other. The wooden bowl in my hands, the paper mâché bowl in my lap, both carrying stories of who we were and who we became. Both reminding me that color has a way of returning, sometimes through the hands of the child who grew up watching me lose it, and then spent his life giving it back.

The memory settled softly around me, like dust drifting back into place. I set the paper mâché bowl aside and looked again at the wooden one in my hands, feeling the weight of both stories at once. Something inside me eased, touched by a tenderness I couldn't quite name—a sense of being connected to Greg in a way that felt both old and newly understood. And in that quiet moment, the only thing that felt right was to reach for my phone.

I texted him immediately, trying to put my emotions into words. "My eyes filled with tears as I opened the box that came today. The bowl is so beautiful, and I love it."

"I'm glad you like it, Mom," he replied. "It's not perfect, but I always liked that one. It's been in my office on my shelf for several years. I figured it could use a better home, so I put a fresh coat of oil on it. It's birch wood that I burned and polished."

I told him that when we'd visited him in April, I had almost asked if I could have one of his "throwaway" projects I'd seen in the garage—the ones he felt weren't worthy of gracing someone's table or sitting on a bookshelf. I had imagined his wooden pieces sparking more conversation than the book titles beside them. But there had been too much going on back then, so I let the thought pass.

"They all mean so much to me," I told him now. "Even the so-called imperfect ones. Thank you so much, Greg. I will cherish it."

"The days of the season slipped by quickly, bringing us to Christmas at last." This year, Greg's family decided to forgo their usual tradition of bringing home a live Christmas tree to plant in their yard after the holiday. Instead, they spent a peaceful day together at home, choosing rest and calm over celebration. They opened the few small packages they had—some wrapped, some still in their Amazon boxes—and simply let the day be what it was.

He called a few hours later, mindful of the three-hour time difference.

"No tree this year, Greg?"

"No, none of us are into it. We just needed a peaceful day."

His words settled into me with a kind of familiarity. I understood the need for quiet, for stepping away from traditions when life has stripped them of their meaning.

A peaceful day can feel like a gift when life has been chaotic and overwhelming. Sometimes creating a pocket of serenity together holds more meaning than any tradition ever could. I used to tell my counseling clients the same thing when they were grieving or navigating difficult seasons. His quiet Christmas stirred memories of my own first holiday after losing my father.

"Do something different," I would say. "Create a new tradition. Sit in stillness, or go to the movies, or walk on the beach."

Anything is better than trying to force an old ritual onto a life that has been turned upside down.

I learned that when I was thirteen. My dad was killed in an industrial accident on October 1st, and everyone insisted Mom should carry on with the holidays as if nothing had changed. Dayna, my eighteen-year-old sister, had married just two weeks before Dad's accident, but five of us were still at home—my brothers, only four and nine, and my sisters, fourteen and sixteen. The pretense of happiness that year was unbearable. We drifted in different directions, and Mom slipped into a long, heavy sadness she never seemed able to climb out of.

Looking back now, I see that season differently. I used to think it was simply the year everything fell apart, but now I understand it as the year I first saw how impossible it is to hold a family together when grief is pulling at every seam. Mom wasn't trying to quiet us or dim anything bright; she was trying to survive something she didn't have words for. That realization came slowly, over years, but it softened something in me.

When she had that surgery years later and came home, she was good for just a few days before she failed again. A home-visiting nurse came by and asked her about the medicines she was taking. Mom said there was a new one the doctor had prescribed—"something for my stomach," she told her.

"Get it for me, Lynnette. It's right on the counter."

I picked up the bottle and read the label. It wasn't for her stomach at all. It was an antidepressant—and in the quiet between us, she knew that I knew. That small moment told me more than she ever said out loud. It wasn't weakness. It wasn't failure. It was the weight of a life she had carried alone for far too long.

So when Greg and his family chose a quiet Christmas, it made sense to me. Stillness can be its own kind of mercy. Sometimes the bravest thing a person can do is step away from the noise and let the day be gentle.

Greg was off work for several days between Christmas and New Year's, a much-needed break while the plant shut down for renovations. But the time off didn't lift anything in him. I found myself calling more often, letting the phone ring longer than usual, waiting for the click of his voice. Sometimes it didn't come. A few minutes later the screen would light up with a short text—"Sorry. Can't talk."

When he did answer, there was a long breath before he spoke, as if he had to gather himself just to say hello. His words came slowly, spaced out, the way someone talks when they're trying not to let anything crack open. Sometimes he paused so long between sentences that I thought the call had dropped. Other times I could hear him shift, or swallow, or exhale through his nose—small sounds that told me more than anything he said out loud.

He wasn't hiding from me. He was just tired in a way that lived inside his voice. He was probably tired of me asking, "How's it going?" and just as tired of having to answer, "not good."

I called him on the afternoon of New Year's Eve because we were heading out to our community dance later that night. He felt terrible, and severe back pain had immobilized him. I've always believed that illness finds the tender places—the parts of us already worn thin. Greg's lifelong diabetes had put his eyes at risk, and years earlier he had injured his back badly enough to require emergency surgery.

Without steady attention to self-care, he became vulnerable to misalignment, and chronic pain followed him like a shadow. I know how easily severe pain can dull a person's ability to make choices in their own best interest. Illness, fatigue, discouragement—they can pull anyone down to the point of not caring.

With how much pain he was in, I gently suggested a warm bath, hoping it might ease things even a little.

"Do you have any Epsom salts? And some lavender essential oil?"

"Oh, yeah. I've got some. I tried a bath before, but it barely took the edge off. Dr. H said I didn't use enough salt. I'll try again when we get off the phone."

His voice was so flat and tired it seemed the call might end quickly. But things shifted when his dad spoke—steady, practical, the way he always was.

"Greg," he said, "you're doing better than you think." A pause. "You're talking more. You're getting out with Murdoch again. That's progress."

Greg exhaled. "I know. It just doesn't feel like it."

His father didn't soften his tone—he never did—but there was a quiet certainty in it.

"Doesn't matter how it feels. It's still true."

I stepped in then, my voice warmer, more coaxing.

"Greg, remember what Dr. H said. Your recovery will take one to two years. It's only been a couple of months. You're allowed to feel tired. Just be gentle with yourself."

His father added, "You're not where you were last year. Not even close."

I continued, "Try the bath again. Add more salt this time—three or four cups, not just a handful. Let the heat work on your back. And when you get out, wrap up in something warm. Give your body a chance to settle."

Greg's voice softened just a little. "Okay. I'll try it."

Greg and his father could always fall into long, animated conversations about motors, engines, electrical problems, and cars—old or new, it didn't matter. They had rebuilt a couple of classic antique cars when Greg was a teenager and even won awards at local shows. These days they could just as easily talk about EVs and hybrids. That was their language.

I didn't have the knowledge or interest to join those conversations, so I focused on the self-care side of things, trying to nudge Greg toward choices that might lift his spirits. I reminded him of the things he used to love.

"Get some of your old albums out and listen to music."

He wasn't up for many of his physical hobbies, but music was still within reach. He'd collected albums since he was a teenager—hundreds of them—and he always insisted that records sounded better than anything digital. He still believed that.

Greg also played guitar and had been in a band when he was younger. I know he still has several guitars, though I'm not sure whether making music still resonates with him the way it once did. Sometimes he just needs a reminder. On second thought, sometimes all of us do. We all need to be nudged toward the things that comfort us, the things that soothe.

I leaned back and closed my eyes. For a moment, I drifted back in time, seeing ten-year-old Greg and me dancing around the living room, laughing as we moved to the jazzy, upbeat organ music his dad played while swaying back and forth. Those were glorious memories.

As our call wound down, a familiar mix of worry and tenderness settled over me—feelings that had followed so much of this past year. Greg was still fighting—some days with determination, other days with whatever scraps of energy he could gather. But he was fighting. And even in his exhaustion, even in the setbacks and the pain, there were glimmers of the man he had been and the man he was becoming.

I held onto that as we said goodnight. His recovery wasn't steady, but it was real. There was movement. There was effort. There was hope. And sometimes, that has to be enough.

As the quiet settled around me, my mind drifted back to the music that once filled our living room—the way sound could lift us, carry us, soothe us. It still could, even now, tucked away like a familiar record waiting to be pulled from its sleeve and set gently on the turntable.

Life had changed in ways none of us could have predicted, but that memory reminded me that comfort doesn't vanish; it simply shifts shape. Sometimes it arrives in a song. Sometimes it arrives in a wooden bowl—one Greg had turned years ago, dusted off, polished, and oiled again in 2025. It sat on my table now, warm in color and weight, a quiet reminder that even when life feels splintered, something beautiful can still be shaped from what remains.

I picked up the bowl, running my hands over its smooth surface, my fingers tracing the rougher edges of his carved initials on the bottom—GW. The contrast felt like him somehow, the polished and the unfinished living side by side. I held it for a long moment, letting its warmth settle into my palms, the grain catching the light in soft, shifting patterns. Outside, the year was turning. Inside, the bowl rested in my hands—solid, imperfect, still becoming.

The paper mâché bowl sits on a shelf across the room now, its wild colors catching the light. For years I thought it was only a relic of who I used to be, but I see it differently these days. Greg was the child who wore the bright clothes and the crazy hats, the one who reminded me—without ever knowing it—that I didn't have to stay folded in on myself forever.

I'm not the girl who hides her hot pink dress anymore. I'm the woman who's wearing it to the

Valentine's dance next week. The one who walked onstage last night in her faux leopard-skinned pants and ridiculous hat, brave and loud and fully myself. It's taken me a long time to understand the things that shaped me.

And somewhere in that understanding, I keep returning to the gift my mother left me. Before she died, she changed her will so her little home in Florida would come to Al and me. "You'll love it here someday," she said. I couldn't see it then—I wasn't even old enough to live in a 55-plus community—but she was right. When we finally moved here, something in me began to unfold again. Valleydale gave me back the parts of myself I lost at thirteen: the color, the boldness, the costumes, the laughter, and the confidence. I think, in her own way, my mother knew she was giving me a place where I could come back to life.

Both bowls sit where I can see them. His, turned in a season of possibility. Mine, made in a season when my color had already dimmed, though I didn't yet know how to name the loss. The story on that bowl held truths I couldn't see then—the light that visited me, and the ally I wrote about, knowing even then that it was Greg, though I couldn't yet accept the gift of what he reflected back to me. He was the one who mirrored back the brightness I'd misplaced, long before I was ready to claim it. Only now, through writing this memoir, do I see how our gifts intertwined. They were never just objects. They were the map.

They remind me that color doesn't vanish. It waits. It waits in memory, in the people who love us, in the parts of ourselves we set aside and eventually find again. It waits in the gifts we give without knowing why, and in the ones we finally learn how to receive.

I've reclaimed my color—not all at once, and not without grief, but piece by piece, the way light returns after a long winter. And as I look at Greg's bowl—warm in my hands, imperfect and beautiful—I feel the quiet truth of it settle in me. Healing isn't a straight line. But color returns.

And I hope, in his own time, Greg will reclaim his too.

CHAPTER EIGHTEEN

Hope in the Hard Places

Greg's journey has carried him from a place of deep despair to a space where hope has begun to take root. Recovery, he was learning, moves more like a piece turning on a lathe—uneven in places, slow in others, shaped gradually rather than all at once. And just as he used to say about his wooden bowls, "It's not perfect," but that never meant it wasn't becoming something worth keeping. Healing doesn't follow a single path or a predictable timeline.

Bartonella fought back with stubborn persistence, yet Greg's strength remained the more powerful force. What he needed most were steady, uncomplicated reminders of that strength— reminders of his courage as he navigated a healthcare system that lacked the resources, knowledge, or compassion to help him. And more than that, he needed those reminders on the days when the slow pace of recovery left him discouraged.

A few months earlier, Greg had called with a strange edge in his voice.

"Mom… did you pay one of my hospital bills?"

"No," I said, already bracing. "Why? What happened?"

"There was this seven-thousand-dollar charge. It's just… gone." He paused. "Like it evaporated."

I tried to lighten the moment. "Well, it definitely wasn't me."

He let out a short laugh, but I could still hear the uncertainty underneath. "I don't know whether to feel relieved or freaked out," he said. "It's just… weird."

"I get it," I said. "But maybe take the win for tonight."

He exhaled, long and tired. "Yeah. I guess I needed one."

After we hung up, I sat with the strangeness of it—how a bill that could crush him financially could also vanish without explanation. It shouldn't work that way. No one should have to celebrate a clerical error just to breathe for a night. And the truth was, we never did find out what happened to that charge. It was just one more oddity in a long list of things that didn't make sense during those months, a brief moment of relief in a system that rarely offered any.

Later, when the house was quiet, I sat at the kitchen table scrolling through Bartonella case studies. Story after story echoed ours—families drained, dismissed, misdiagnosed. I kept hoping to find one person who got help without losing their savings or their sanity. I didn't. The weight of it pressed in: this wasn't just Greg's fight. It was the fight of anyone whose illness didn't fit neatly into a diagnostic box.

When an illness is invisible, misunderstood, or unexplained, the person living with it carries not only the physical burden but also the emotional weight of not being believed, not being supported, and not being seen. That combination can be deeply isolating. It's one thing to fight a condition with a clear diagnosis and a clear path forward; it's another to fight in the dark, trying to convince others—and sometimes even yourself—that your pain is real.

Through all of this, my hope was simple: that Greg would keep nurturing the small shoots of optimism taking root in him. Life was still unpredictable, but he was beginning to meet it with a steadier heart.

Somewhere in those months, a quiet realization settled in. What matters most is compassionate, patient-centered care. Even when answers are elusive, people deserve validation and continuity—sometimes recognition alone is a lifeline.

Greg follows several forums about chronic Lyme, Bartonella, and related vector-borne diseases, and it saddens him to see the desperation of people searching for answers.

"So many people are where I was a year ago."

"That's sad, Greg. Do you chime in?"

"No. I don't have the answers either, and I'm not well enough to invest myself in other people's struggles yet. It's such an individual journey."

Even as he watched others struggle, he was slowly reclaiming pieces of his own life.

Just yesterday, he texted me a picture of a "new" dishwasher—a free one he spotted on his way home from work. He was excited, almost proud, running it through cycles to clean it up. For months, he hadn't had the strength, energy, or even the spare money to replace the one that had died. I had wanted so badly to swoop in and fix it for him, to call Home Depot and have a new one delivered and installed without him lifting a finger.

That urge to rescue him lived just under my skin. But early on, his dad and I agreed that while we would fully support his medical care, we couldn't step in to solve every practical problem. Greg needed space to rebuild his own life, in his own way. And this time, he did. He lifted it, hauled it home in the open hatch of his Honda Fit, took a chance on it, and made it work. It was just a dishwasher, but it felt like something more—a small, ordinary victory that signaled his capacity returning, his confidence flickering back to life. His excitement came through the text, and for the first time in a long while, something shifted in me too.

And then another moment arrived, one that reached back to the months when everything felt like it was slipping away.

When I visited Washington that spring, the yard told its own story—overgrown grass, sagging outbuildings, vehicles sitting untouched in the rain. One afternoon, a man pulled up and asked about the white Chevy pickup parked near the garage. He said he'd been driving by for weeks and noticed it hadn't moved. Would I consider selling it?

"Oh, it's not mine," I said. "I'll go ask my son."

For a moment, I thought it might be a small blessing for Greg, a way to bring in a little extra money. I went inside to ask him. He was resting in his recliner—the only real piece of furniture left in the living room besides one other chair. The leather couch we'd given them when we moved had probably been hauled to the dump by then, long since worn down by Maple and Mona, both Great Pyrenees mixes, who still thought they were lap dogs.

"Greg, someone wants to buy the truck," I said. "Do you want to sell it?"

He didn't hesitate. "No. I'll get back to it someday."

There was no arguing with that kind of certainty, even though the truck had been sitting untouched for years. I told the man it wasn't for sale and watched him drive away, thinking the pickup would probably end up in a junkyard someday, another casualty of the life Greg had been forced to set aside.

But just last week, Greg called me, his voice bright in a way I hadn't heard in so long. He'd jump-started the battery, evicted a mouse from the glove box, and the one-ton Chevy pickup roared back to life.

Meagan was happy too—it meant she could finally haul the free wood chips she'd been wanting for the garden she was trying to revive.

It wasn't just a truck starting.

It was Greg starting.

Another small, stubborn victory—proof that the parts of himself he thought he'd lost were still waiting for him.

A few days later, I found myself thinking about Murdoch. During our visit to Washington, he had spent most of his time tucked away in his room, quiet and self-contained, navigating more than any fourteen-year-old should have to carry. But one afternoon, after we picked Greg up from work, Murdoch came downstairs and stood in front of me—tall, gentle, hesitant.

"Grandma… could we go to the thrift store?"

It was such a small question, but it felt like a door opening. "Of course, Doc," I said. "Let's check with your dad and Grandpa, and we'll meet your mom after."

And that's exactly what we did. He wandered the aisles with a kind of quiet delight, choosing treasures, letting himself enjoy something simple. It was an ordinary outing, but it felt like another light in the dark—a moment of connection I held onto long after we drove home.

None of us could have predicted that Smokey—the stray kitten we rescued years ago and who became part of our family—might have played a role in what followed with Greg's health. That possibility only surfaced in hindsight, long after Greg became sick. Whether he was the beginning of it or just one piece of a larger puzzle, we couldn't know. What we did know was that the illness that took hold reshaped everything.

Yet each new day brings the possibility of incremental healing and the hope that, with determination and the support of those who care, Greg can reclaim a sense of normalcy. When I spoke with him today, his voice was strong, and he said his brain felt sharper and his thinking clearer.

"My thoughts are more coherent, and I have more clarity." "Also, my eyes seem better, but my back is killing me."

I shared my theory about how the bacteria seemed to target the most vulnerable places in his body.

"Yeah, you're probably right, Mom."

"Just be kind to yourself. Simple movements, gentle exercise, hot baths."

"Thanks, Mom. I'll do that."

Greg's journey has shown me how quickly life can tilt, how joy and hardship can sit side by side, shaping us in ways we never expect.

Even now, with uncertainty still present, a sense of hope is taking shape as understanding grows and new possibilities emerge. Greg's story is not one of easy answers or quick recoveries. It is a story of endurance—of a man who refused to disappear into the illness that tried to claim him. It is a story of a family learning to listen, to trust, and to let go of the illusion that we can control the path of someone we love.

As winter softened into the promise of spring, Greg's voice carried a new steadiness, a quiet confidence that had been missing for far too long. And in that moment, I realized that healing isn't measured in milestones or timelines. It's measured in the return of a laugh, the clarity of a thought, the courage to imagine a future again. Sometimes it's even measured in the small, ordinary victories he claims on his own—the ones I once would have rushed to claim for him.

He is still healing. We all are. But momentum was returning—unmistakable.

As we said goodbye, he told me he hoped to fly again in the spring. It was a simple statement, but it carried the weight of everything he had fought for.

"I'll see you in the spring, Mom."

"You think you're going to be able to fly again soon?"

"That's the goal, Mom."

I felt a faint echo of his eight-year-old voice, the one that once steadied me on a busy road. *Don't worry, Mom, it will be okay.* I let the memory settle inside me, offering him the same reassurance now, even if only in my heart.

Those words stayed with me—not as a promise, but as a direction to lean toward life again. Toward possibility. Toward the quiet belief that even in an uncertain world, hope can take root and grow.

There are moments in life when the ordinary becomes sacred—a text, a breath, a quiet exchange that steadies the heart. This chapter of our lives was full of those moments, small lights in a long stretch of darkness. Some were as simple as a picture of a free dishwasher, a flicker of excitement that told me more about his healing than any lab result ever could. Those lights reminded me of another night long ago, when I crawled into a dark culvert searching for a fragile life that refused to give up. I didn't know then that I would one day follow that glow again—this time for my son.

And in those small lights, I felt the quiet truth that love and hope walk beside us, even when the path is dark. For now, that was enough—a beginning, not an ending.

AUTHORS NOTE

Greg, this story begins in the quiet hours when worry keeps me awake and love refuses to let me look away. I write it to trace the shape of what you are enduring, but also to honor the light you carry through the darkest corridors of your life. You are walking a path no one can walk for you, yet every step echoes in my own heart.

There are days when your strength is a whisper, days when hope feels thin as breath—yet still you move forward. Still you search. Still you hold on. Watching you teaches me that resilience is not loud or heroic; sometimes it is simply the act of rising again, even when the world feels unbearably heavy.

If you ever read these pages, I hope you feel the love threaded through every line, the kind that stretches across miles and years and uncertainty. I hope you see the man you are becoming in the midst of everything that tries to break you.

You are the quiet miracle at the center of this story—and the reason it is worth telling. Through you, I am learning that even the hardest places can become a path toward healing.

I don't know how long this road will be for you, Greg, or what shape your healing will ultimately take. What I do know is that you have never walked it alone. Every step you take—the faltering ones, the brave ones, the ones you don't think you can manage—reveals a strength that continues to humble me. This story isn't written from the safety of an ending; it's written from the middle, where fear and hope live side by side. And even here, in the unfinished places, I watch you rise again and again, carrying a light that refuses to go out.

And if the road ahead remains uncertain, then we will meet it the way we always have—with hope held gently in our hands, lighting the hard places one step at a time.

Further Reading & Resources

During the years I spent trying to understand what was happening to my son, I read everything I could find—scientific papers, case reports, personal essays, and the stories of other families who had walked their own bewildering paths through vector-borne illness. None of these materials offered simple answers, but each one helped me see a little more of the landscape we were navigating.

The following books, articles, and resources are not endorsements or conclusions. They are simply the pieces of information that shaped my understanding during a time of searching, learning, and trying to make sense of a complex medical journey. Readers who wish to explore further may find this a helpful place to begin.

1. Bartonella-Specific Narratives & Case Stories

These stories focus directly on Bartonella and offer insight into the lived experience of individuals and families confronting this infection. One is a full-length memoir; one is a condensed version written for an advocacy organization.

Bell, N. D. (2021). What Lurks in the Woods:
    Struggle and Hope in the Midst of Chronic
    Illness. A memoir chronicling one family's
    journey through a complex, ultimately fatal
    case of Bartonella infection.

Bell, N. D. (2021). Bartonella: The Beast Within.
    Project Lyme. A condensed article based
    on the same story as What Lurks in the
    Woods, written for a general audience.

Newby, K. (2022). Swamp Boy – Medical Mystery:
    A Story About Bartonella and Mental
    Illness. Epic Magazine. A long-form
    narrative exploring a young man's struggle
    with severe neuropsychiatric symptoms
    later linked to Bartonella.

2. Readable Case Studies & Scientific Articles

These publications are scientific in nature but
accessible to non-specialists. They helped me
understand the diagnostic challenges, symptom
variability, and emerging research surrounding
Bartonella.

Dempsey, T. Vector-Borne Infections: Focus on
    Bartonella.
    https://drtaniadempsey.com/vector-
    borne-infections-focus-on-bartonella/

Schaller, J., Burkland, G. A., & Langhoff, P. J. (2007). Do Bartonella Infections Cause Agitation, Panic Disorder, and Treatment-Resistant Depression? Medscape General Medicine, 9(3):54.

Peake, T. (2020). Study: Bartonella Infection Associated with Psychiatric Symptoms and Skin Lesions. North Carolina State University.

Breitschwerdt, E., Bradley, J., Maggi, R., Lashnits, E., & Reicherter, P. (2020). Bartonella-Associated Cutaneous Lesions (BACL) in People with Neuropsychiatric Symptoms. Pathogens. DOI: 10.3390/pathogens9121023

Breitschwerdt, E., Greenberg, R., Maggi, R., Mozayeni, R., Lewis, A., & Bradley, J. (2019). Bartonella henselae Bloodstream Infection in a Boy with Pediatric Acute-Onset Neuropsychiatric Syndrome. DOI: 10.1177/1179573519832014

Moresco, A. (2025). Pathobiome Perspectives: How Bartonella Hijacks the Brain's Immune System. LymeDisease.org

Selected Case Reports (General-Audience Friendly):

Bartonella henselae Infection Presenting With Neuroretinitis (American Journal of Ophthalmology)

Bartonella Infection Mimicking Autoimmune Disease (BMJ Case Reports)

Pediatric Bartonella Neuropsychiatric Case Reports (Journal of Central Nervous System Disease)

3. Broader Memoirs & Narratives Involving Vector-Borne Illness

These books are not exclusively about Bartonella, but they include Bartonella as part of the broader picture of chronic vector-borne disease. They offer readers a sense of the many different paths people take when confronting complex, poorly understood illnesses.

Phillips, S., MD & Parish, D. (2020). Chronic. A narrative driven exploration of chronic vector-borne illness, including patient stories involving Bartonella.

Spector, N., MD. Gone in a Heartbeat. A physician's personal account of misdiagnosed vector-borne illness; Bartonella appears in the broader context.

Douthat, R. The Deep Places. A memoir about chronic illness and the search for answers; includes discussion of co-infections.

Dennis, L. Lyme Madness. A parent's account of advocating for her son through complex illness; Bartonella is part of the narrative landscape.

4. Related Medical Research

These studies explore broader biological mechanisms—including immune, neurological, and vascular pathways—that may overlap with symptoms seen in vector-borne illness. They are included here because they helped me understand how complex and interconnected these conditions can be.

Coucha, M., Abdelsaid, M., & Bolduc, D. (2022). *The Impact of COVID-19 Spike Protein on the Retinal Microvascular Environment.* Investigative Ophthalmology & Visual Science.

Singh, P. K., Balendiran, V., Monu, M., Ahmad, F., & Olson, R. (2024). *COVID-19 Virus*

Could Damage Vision. University of Missouri School of Medicine.

5. Organizations & Educational Resources

These organizations offer information, support, and research related to Bartonella, vector-borne illness, and chronic complex conditions.

Project Lyme — https://projectlyme.org

LymeDisease.org — https://www.lymedisease.org

Global Lyme Alliance —
> https://www.globallymealliance.org

Columbia University Lyme & Tick-Borne Diseases Research Center —
> https://www.columbia-lyme.org

Bartonella Research and Advocacy Network (BRAN) —
> https://www.bartonellaresearch.com

North Carolina State University – Intracellular Pathogens Research Laboratory —
> https://cvm.ncsu.edu

A Note on How to Approach These Materials

These readings vary widely—some are scientific, some are deeply personal, and some sit somewhere in between. They reflect the uncertainty, debate, and evolving research that surround Bartonella and other vector-borne illnesses. I encourage readers to approach them with curiosity rather than fear, and with the understanding that no single study or story captures the full picture. What they offer is perspective: glimpses into the many different ways people make sense of illness, healing, and the long road in between.

About the Author

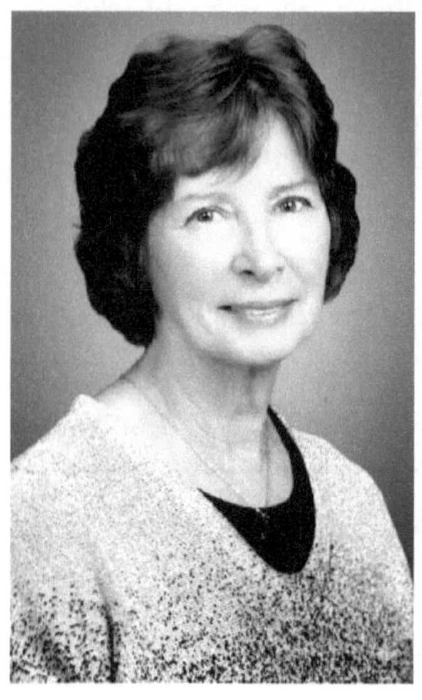

Lynnette M. Wheeler spends her winters in
Zephyrhills, Florida, and her summers on Lake
Embden in Maine—places that have shaped her
love of community, nature, and quiet reflection.
For thirty years, she worked as a psychotherapist,
guiding others through their own seasons of
struggle and resilience. She also taught Psychology
and Sociology of Marriage and Family at
community colleges, sharing her passion for

understanding the human experience with students of all ages.

A lifelong lover of movement, she found joy in pickleball, paddleboarding, and an active lifestyle—until life asked her to slow down and listen more deeply. When injury temporarily closed those physical doors, she returned to writing, a passion she had carried since childhood and rediscovered with renewed devotion during the pandemic.

She is the author of *Missy Lynn's Extraordinary Journey*, its sequel *Missy Lynn Returns*, and *A Walk of Faith—A Poetic Journey Through Life*. She has also co-authored several books with her close friend, Dr. George McGuire. Lynnette now serves as a social club director in her community and continues to find meaning in connection, service, and creative expression. She has been married for forty-eight years.

This memoir grew from a mother's love and a desire to honor her son Greg's courage as he navigated a bewildering and often invisible illness. What began as a search for answers became a journey of acceptance, gratitude, and spiritual awareness. Through Greg's struggle, she learned that the greatest lessons rarely come from triumph, but from the willingness to endure, to stay connected, and to keep moving forward when life asks more of us than we ever imagined.

She wrote this book to give voice to those living with hidden illnesses, to shed light on experiences often dismissed or misunderstood, and to remind others that even in the darkest seasons, there is always a path—however faint—leading back toward hope. Above all, she wrote it so Greg would never feel alone or abandoned, and so others walking similar paths might feel seen.